The Yoga of Right Diet

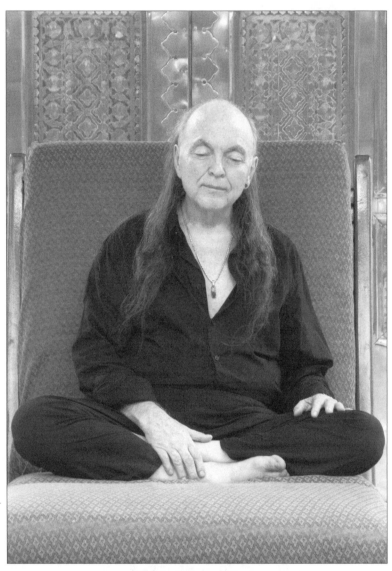

The Avataric Great Sage,
ADI DA SAMRAJ

The
Yoga
of
Right Diet

An Intelligent Approach
to Dietary Practice
That Supports Communion with
the Living Divine Reality

by
The Avataric Great Sage,
ADI DA SAMRAJ

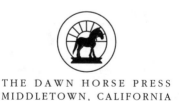

THE DAWN HORSE PRESS
MIDDLETOWN, CALIFORNIA

NOTE TO THE READER

All who study the Way of Adidam or take up its practice should remember that they are responding to a Call to become responsible for themselves. They should understand that they, not Avatar Adi Da Samraj or others, are responsible for any decision they make or action they take in the course of their lives of study or practice.

The devotional, Spiritual, functional, practical, relational, and cultural practices and disciplines referred to in this book are appropriate and natural practices that are voluntarily and progressively adopted by members of the practicing congregations of Adidam (as appropriate to the personal circumstance of each individual). The diet and health approach outlined in this book is one such practical discipline. Although anyone may find these practices useful and beneficial, they are not presented as advice or recommendations to the general reader or to anyone who is not a member of one of the practicing congregations of Adidam. And nothing in this book is intended as a diagnosis, prescription, or recommended treatment or cure for any specific "problem", whether medical, emotional, psychological, social, or Spiritual. One should apply a particular program of treatment, prevention, cure, or general health only in consultation with a licensed physician or other qualified professional.

The Yoga of Right Diet is formally authorized for publication by the Ruchira Sannyasin Order of Adidam Ruchiradam. (The Ruchira Sannyasin Order of Adidam Ruchiradam is the senior Cultural Authority within the formal gathering of formally acknowledged devotees of the Avataric Great Sage, Adi Da Samraj.)

CONTENTS

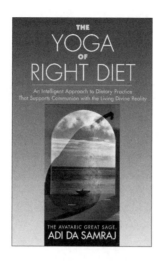

ABOUT THE COVER

Throughout His Life, Avatar Adi Da Samraj has worked to develop means—both literary and artistic—of communicating the True Nature of Reality. He approaches the creation of His literary and artistic works as a process of Revealing What Reality Is and how Its True Nature can be Realized.

For the cover of *The Yoga of Right Diet*, Avatar Adi Da has chosen an image He created in 2003 (*2003_078_12*). This image was created entirely in-camera, by means of multiple exposure.

Examples of the artwork of Adi Da Samraj, together with discussions of His artwork and His own statements about it, may be seen online at:

www.daplastique.com

INTRODUCTION

Y ou are about to read several Talks and Essays by the Avataric Great Sage, Adi Da Samraj. What you will find is not the usual information regarding health, but rather a unique description of diet and healing from a "point of view" that is entirely "radical".

Most men and women look to feel good—understandably so. They go about this via diverse means, using many methods and disciplines in order to pursue their goal. Some find improvements, some fewer numbers are lucky to attain a state that feels really good, but a great many are burdened by chronic problems that make health seem to be very elusive indeed.

Adi Da Samraj's approach to the matter of diet and health is both straightforward and profound. He says that true "food" is Reality Itself, and that true health is "about sustenance, about love, and not really about conventional matters of diet and health". Thus, to truly be healthy, one must locate the True Source-Condition of all that appears, and it is from there that healing can occur. One must, of course, use practical means available for healing, and diet is key among such means. But one starts with Reality and one's Communion with Reality—and, then, practical health matters are dealt with from this starting point.

For the body to be in touch with the Divine Source-Condition, one must have prepared it as a vehicle fit for such Communion, free from as many obstructions as possible. Therefore, one eats a diet that is pure and allows the body to be in its native condition—which is free of toxicity and enervation. The "minimum-optimum diet" is what Adi Da Samraj recommends to His devotees. This diet makes it easy to assimilate nutrients without overtaxing the body's metabolic systems, and it also makes it easy to eliminate what is not needed (or the breakdown products of that metabolism).

As Adi Da Samraj says in this book, there is no particular diet that is right for everyone. Right diet is a matter that must be determined on an individual basis. However, for the great majority of people, the optimal diet turns out to be one that is predominantly raw, with many variations contained in this raw spectrum. Others find it necessary to eat some portion of cooked foods. All of this is based on the "radical" nature of true healing—which is, fundamentally, Communion with the Source, or Reality, or Real God. Thus, the real purpose of right diet is not necessarily to feel good, but rather to prepare the body for this Communion. Of course, an inevitable product of the minimum-optimum diet is improved health, but this is a secondary aspect—not the goal of right dietary practice.

Avatar Adi Da's recommendations relative to diet are a fundamental part of His unique approach to the matter of "radical" healing. Generally, when people do not feel well, they try to diagnose their ills either on their own or by seeking professional help (whether from conventional doctors or from naturally oriented healers). Such a method boils down to making an objective assessment of what is wrong by various forms of testing—such as blood tests, x-rays, and so forth. This approach is effective for some problems—and necessary particularly with acute trauma and catastrophic medical and surgical emergencies. And the same basic approach is also useful for many other problems, in order to have some idea how to approach the malady at hand. However, the hope in this methodology is that once the "problem" is diagnosed, the patient can take a substance or substances that will result in a "cure". Such is the "substance approach" to healing. In a great many cases, no objective diagnosis is found, even after exhaustive testing. What is one to do next?

As an alternative to the "substance approach", Adi Da Samraj recommends a "systems approach", which allows the body to deal with whatever problem is present, at its root, without even knowing the name of the illness. Thus, many people with symptoms that are otherwise difficult to treat can be cured or helped by adapting the body to this approach, which is essentially done via fasting and raw diet. These means allow the body to purify and then regenerate itself. In the following readings, you will find the basic principles that Adi Da Samraj Teaches regarding right diet and the right use of periodic fasting, as basic means of this "systems approach" to healing.

I sincerely hope that the Wisdom communicated in the following Essays and Talks will cause in you a recognition of the true nature of life, diet, and health—and that you will want to study more of Adi Da Samraj's Teaching and, more importantly, learn more about the great gift of relationship to the Avataric Great Sage, Adi Da Samraj.

Charles Seage, MD
May 2006

The Avataric Great Sage,
Adi Da Samraj

Thousands of people have discovered the Truth for Real when they encountered the Words of Avatar Adi Da Samraj. And Truth Itself is the Gift that Avatar Adi Da Samraj wishes to Offer to you.

Avatar Adi Da's entire Life—starting with His birth on Long Island, New York, in 1939—has been devoted to Communicating the Truth to others. He now Offers His full Communication of Truth in a series of books known as His "Source-Texts". The Essays and Talks in this book are excerpted from those "Source-Texts". And those "Source-Texts", taken together, are His complete Revelation of the Way He Offers to all—the religion of Adidam.

All of Avatar Adi Da's Words are an invitation to consider the Truth of Reality. And, even more than that, all of Avatar Adi Da's Words are an invitation to enter into a real and profound Spiritual relationship with Him—for He has always said, "I Offer you a relationship, not a technique."

Many who have started by reading Avatar Adi Da's Words have gone on to enter into this relationship as His formal devotees. And they have done so because they made the most amazing discovery of their lives:

Avatar Adi Da Samraj is not merely a highly developed human being. He is able to speak the Truth for Real because He is Himself the Living Divine Truth, Appearing on earth in a human body. In other words, He is the Eternal Real God—not the "Creator-God" of traditional religion, but the Very Divine Heart of Reality Itself—Appearing bodily for a time in our midst. He is the One Whom beings have prayed to and hoped for throughout the ages—the Promised and long-Awaited God-Man to come.

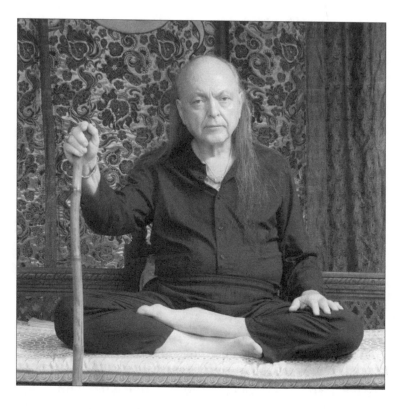

Avatar Adi Da Samraj does not ask you to merely <u>believe</u> this about Him. He simply invites you to come to know Him—by freely considering His Words, and fully feeling their impact on your life and your heart. ■

The Yoga of Right Diet

Renouncing the Search for the Edible Deity

A Talk by
Avatar Adi Da Samraj

1.

AVATAR ADI DA SAMRAJ: Human beings chronically regard their individuation, their birth, their mere bodily existence, to be a form of separation, and they use such events as coming out of the womb and the conflicts of childhood to elaborate this fundamental philosophical "point of view". The inherent vulnerability of apparently independent existence is a shock, and the born person reflects on all experience—even the most primitive movements in the womb—as a kind of rejection. When such a person looks out into the universe, he or she feels insulted, rejected, unloved—and so makes philosophy of apparent independence.

The primal event of suffering is not any circumstance that happens to you, nor an event within your objective experience. It is not anything that you conceive to exist in relation to you, or over against you. The primal event of suffering <u>is</u> you—and your suffering is not a matter of any

<u>actual</u> separation from everything else. Rather, the primal event of your suffering is your own (apparently) independent existence. On the basis of presuming your independent existence, you <u>interpret</u> the present event as separation. That interpretation is your first philosophical gesture, the first time that you say or feel "you do not love me".

Fundamentally, your experiences in particular relationships do not communicate to you that you are not loved. It is factually true that some people do not love you—but, regardless of that ordinary fact, you are simply, always, and already philosophically disposed to feel that you are not loved. That you are not loved is your interpretation of existence—not on the basis of any particular relational experience you have had with other human beings, but on the basis of your (apparent) independent bodily existence itself. Your sense of independent bodily existence <u>means</u> separation to you—but that is an interpretation, not a "reality". When you become a truly mature adult human being, then you stop interpreting the universe as a form of rejection, as a great "parent" from whose company you have been expelled, under whose domination you live, and who has rejected you and does not love you. Everyone is born into the ordinary condition of apparent bodily independence—and everyone interprets that condition as rejection, as "you do not love me".

You are fundamentally disposed to be contracted in your feeling. That disposition is not really the result of your experience, whatever your experience may have been. That disposition may be <u>reinforced</u> by means of your day to day experience, but that disposition is not the <u>result</u> of experience. That disposition is your philosophy, your "point of view". It is the presumption you make in the instant that you acknowledge your functional (bodily) independence. Thus, the bodily independent "I/me" is felt as "you do not love me"—and, therefore, the bodily independent "I/me" lives as unlove, as "I do not love you". Such unlove remains your disposition until you become awakened from the sleep of "vital shock",[*1] from the shock of birth—not the birth trauma in the purely physiological sense, but the acknowledgement of bodily independence, the steady and increasing observation that you are vulnerable, that you are subject to circumstances, that your very existence can apparently depend on circumstances. The more you observe existence in the disposition of vital shock, the more justified you feel in presuming, under all conditions, that "you do not love me".

What is of interest and significance about diet and health is implicit in this metaphysical supposition—which everyone presently lives and, also, by which everyone interprets his or her past. Birth—or the recognition of one's independent bodily existence—is interpreted by you to be separation. It is interpreted by you as an instant, although prolonged through time, in which you are essentially unloved. And all of that interpretation is based on the feeling that you are not sustained. In other words, independent bodily existence is, itself, felt to be separation from the ultimate food-source.

Human beings are mad, then. They are different from the eating gorilla. The eating gorilla finds a cabbage in the jungle, sits down and munches on the cabbage, and is completely benign, completely peaceful. There is nothing threatening, nothing dangerous about this gorilla. The gorilla is not eating anything killed that has an independent consciousness in the ordinary sense—just cabbages, vegetables. If another gorilla comes near, the eating gorilla still has some food, and is (thereby) connected to the food-source. The eating gorilla is not disturbed, as long as the approaching creature shows that he or she is also eating. The eating gorilla is peaceful.

Therefore, the eating gorilla is the image of the true human being. The eating gorilla demonstrates the principle

*Notes to the Text of *The Yoga of Right Diet* appear on pp. 69–82.

16

of true politics, of real human existence—wherein people are always presently connected to Truth, Reality, Happiness, Real (Acausal) God, the Real Food-Source, wherein they are always presuming connection, relationship, "I love you". On the other hand, the gorilla in the desert—or the usual human being—is cut off from the food-source through the presumption of separate existence, the presumption of mortality. The usual human being feels unloved. Such a person is a dangerous beast, in conflict with himself or herself, struggling, looking for a way to be permanently sustained.

All of your conventional efforts in life are searches to be permanently, absolutely, unqualifiedly sustained, to be fed perfectly and eternally, and to be simply happy, kept alive by Whatever put you into existence to begin with. However, until you make your connection with food (or sustenance), you are mad. Since sustenance is scarce, you threaten others. You live like a beast! If you acquire a little bit that sustains you, you become anxious about sustenance and you cannot get enough. You overeat, or you overseek. You are always presuming the logic that you are not sustained, that you are cut off from the source, that you are not loved, that you are separated from that which is capable of (essentially, and permanently, and absolutely) sustaining you. You may get a meal, but where are you going to get the next one? Or even if you can get the next one, how can you live forever?

Ultimately, you must transcend this metaphysics, this philosophy that "I am not loved", that "I am separate from what sustains me". The entire drama of human existence is about precisely this feeling of separation—and that is all.

Rightly engaged, eating is an occasion of meditating on love. When you sit down to eat, you are obliged to meditate on sustenance. If you would consciously approach the entire matter of eating, you must become aware of unlove, of separativeness, of fear, sorrow, anger, guilt, doubt, anxiety—terrible things. In such a condition, there is no way to finish a meal! In your chronic subjectivity, your "Narcissistic"[2] and unloving self-consciousness, you think such negative feelings are true of you. Because you think that such negative feelings are a real and justified experience, you are not sustained by all your eating and all your relations. Yet, you have adapted socially in such a manner that you are willing to accept a vision of mortality and make the best of it. You know that you can eat and continue for a while. You know that you can create circumstances that allow you to continue to live—such that you can eat with relative ease, even though you are, fundamentally, in mortal fear.

Now, there are many ways to approach this entire affair. First of all—in your self-awareness, your self-consciousness, in your acknowledgement of your own functional independence (in the first instant of that acknowledgement, and in every subsequent moment of that acknowledgment)—is it true that you are actually separated from sustenance? To find this out is very important, because everyone simply and mechanically presumes that it is true. The vulnerabilities of childhood reinforce that presumption—as a virtual automaticity. All the habitual social learning of childhood and adolescence that you carry into your later life supports the fundamental metaphysical view that you are unloved, that you are separated from the Absolute That Sustains you, that you are mortal. The more you meditate on being unloved, the less you live as love.

If you allow yourself to feel your actual condition, to feel as your actual condition, to completely feel your condition in this moment, can you discover any separation from anything whatsoever? Are you anything that can be separated, that is separate, that is an "anything" when viewed as a totality?

Such is My essential "Consideration" with you through My Avataric Divine Wisdom-Teaching. If you could simply feel your condition—feel as your condition in this moment, without obstruction, without making an interpretation—then you would no longer be what you are presently being. In that case, you would not be trapped in obstructed feeling-attention and defining yourself, feeling vulnerable, separate, "a" being. You would directly and intuitively discover the Source-Condition in Which you and every thing and every one is arising (without, in any sense, being separated out), in Which you exist Non-conditionally, in Which you are Sustained Absolutely, and in Which you never were (or are) separated from anything.

Thus, reconnecting to your sustenance is a matter of unobstructed feeling-attention, through all your functions, as the entire body-mind—in all your relations, and under all conditions. That is all it is. In that participatory sacrifice of separative and separate self, you are love. You are an expression of the Divine Nature of all things. When you are thus unobstructed, the body-mind itself is love. When you become responsible for the compulsive contraction of feeling-attention in yourself, then you are naturally sustained and a natural sustainer of others. Your humor is restored, and you are released from the desert. You cease to be a beast, a subhuman, maniacal creature—and you become natural, peaceful, pleasant, loving, intimate, humorous. Existence becomes a matter of inherent pleasurableness, not the beastly struggle for the acquisition of experiential pleasure, the temporary attainment of the sense of being sustained. If you live in this manner, you can live a happy and loving and healthy life, an essentially vital life. Although there may be limitations that come upon you through the environmental and human factors around you, essentially you can be the master of your circumstance, at least in your private life.

Love or not—that is all there is to it. If you can come again to the position of loving in the sense that I have just Described—of being sustained and being a sustainer in the natural flow of things—then you will continue to grow, and the very structural dimensions toward which you are experientially disposed will show themselves, auspiciously, in the form of experience. You must be responsible for the effects of those dimensions of the body-mind. You must be responsible in every moment, such that, no matter what arises, the self-contraction[3] is not your destiny, not your disposition in the moment. You must be able to go beyond that contraction—whatever the experience, high or low.

2.

AVATAR ADI DA SAMRAJ: Once you have become truly self-responsible, only then are you truly human. At the point of such self-responsibility, there are some more sophisticated things to be observed about sustenance—about diet and health and gross existence.[4] You observe that, in terms of your conventional (or mechanical) state of existence, you are a very simple process. The entirety of your functional, bodily, conditionally manifested life is, fundamentally, a very simple process—albeit a complicated "play" on a simple process. You are simply reception-and-release. And that binary dynamism, which is epitomized in the cycle of inhalation and exhalation, is also the very foundation of your entire psycho-physical life. The matter of diet and health is simply a matter of applying yourself with intelligence to this dynamic process, to the Law that is this process itself.

Now, how do you stay healthy? By being responsible for reception (or assimilation) and release (or elimination). If you are not so responsible, you become toxic (or unable to release) and enervated (or unable to receive, to be sustained, to assimilate).

The process of adaptation to the Way of Adidam (Which is the heart-practice of the devotional relationship to Me) begins with the ordinary individual who is just a beast in the desert. As My beginning devotee, you respond to Me by devotionally recognizing Me As the Avataric Divine Incarnation of the Inherently Perfect and Self-Evidently Divine Reality in Which you exist, and (also) by observing the primal emotional reaction, the metaphysical presumption of separation and unlove, to the point that you are able to live like the peaceful eating gorilla and (thus) to be human, to be love.

Likewise, as My devotee, you are Called, by Me, to observe the cycle of your existence, in relationship to the great pattern in which you appear—which you have not created, and within which you are totally dependent. The process by which you appear is not within you, nor does it originate in you. You are simply a reflection of a great pattern. That great pattern is expressed everywhere—in the form of all processes, all individuals, all the cycles that are everywhere to be observed. The great process is simply the cycle of reception and release, inhalation and exhalation, assimilation and elimination, activity and rest.

Having come to this point of understanding, how do you become healthy? The practice of right diet and health involves a process of responsible (and progressive) adaptation. That process may, at times, be animated similarly at every meal, or, at other times, differently every day, or even (occasionally) in more dramatic fashion, through fasting or other more rigorously conservative dietary regimes. Nevertheless, the adaptation to the practice of right diet and health is a single process, a process of reception and release.

The failure of health is the failure of the cycle of reception and release. When your health has failed, you have allowed the body-mind to become toxic and enervated. If you take a great amount into yourself that you cannot assimilate, what is not used by the body accumulates in the body. This is true not only of gross food but of all your experience.

The more you become full of accumulations, the more toxic (or "poisoned" in the body and obstructed in feeling-attention) you become, and (consequently) the less energy you represent and the less love you <u>are</u>. Therefore, the discipline of ordinary eating and drinking and managing the body is, most fundamentally, to take conscious responsibility for the cycle of reception and release.

The primary obstruction to your energy in the moment is accumulation, or toxicity. Thus, the first phase in the regaining—or in the ordinary maintenance—of health is purification, or the elimination of toxins, accumulations, and obstructions. This purification is the effect of right practice that you will observe at the level of gross (physical) diet.

Purification is also the initial effect of meditation. Indeed, the foundation stages of Spiritual life are, essentially, a matter of purification. Such purification is not the result of asceticism for its own sake. Such asceticism is a one-sided (and, thus, misguided) effort (or strategy) of purification-<u>only</u>, exhalation-<u>only</u>, or elimination-<u>only</u>. Having gone through a period of purification and release of toxins, one enters into the second phase of true health practice, which is the phase of assimilation, regeneration, and rejuvenation. In this phase, the mechanisms of the body are re-stimulated. It becomes possible to fully engage the receptivity of the body-mind. The entire body-mind participates in this purifying and regenerative process, whereby <u>both</u> reception <u>and</u> release—the eliminative and the assimilative aspects of this single (or entire-body) process—become a matter of responsibility. Thus, right practice of the Way of Adidam addresses the entire body-mind, by becoming responsible for both the purifying (or eliminative) and the regenerative (or assimilative) aspects of the process of the body-mind.

The fundamental principle of health is the balancing of these two natural phases of the life-process—purification and rejuvenation. If either the purification phase or the rejuvenation phase of the cycle becomes exaggerated, the person becomes psycho-physically imbalanced and (therefore) no longer healthy. If your participation in the purification (or eliminative) phase becomes exaggerated, you become enervated, because essential nutrients have been depleted from the system. If you exaggerate the regeneration (or assimilative) phase by consuming more food than the body can easily and quickly use and eliminate, you become toxic.

At times, you must exercise the process of elimination and assimilation with greater intensity than usual—as a treatment regime during a period of illness, or as an annual period of cleansing and revitalization, or (perhaps, occasionally) as a particularly intensive period of purification and rejuvenation. But you must also engage the process of elimination and assimilation daily. You must eat like the gorilla. You must breathe like the gorilla. What you choose to eat should not toxify or enervate you. What you choose to eat, on a daily basis, should be easily assimilated by the body and should be completely satisfying. In other words, your diet should include everything that every part of the entire body needs.

Just so, the body should be easily able to eliminate the unusable portion of the food that it ingests. It should not have to hide waste products in the cells—until, eventually, the wastes emerge as disease. Your eating must (itself) satisfy the Law of your own psycho-physical mechanism—the dual Law of assimilation (or sustenance) and elimination (or purification). Such a Lawful diet must be your daily choice—once you become responsible for yourself, once you understand your True Condition, and once you are (therefore) no longer "mad", like a beast in the desert, but (rather) you are happy.

There are certain substances commonly consumed by human beings which are fundamentally toxifying and enervating—even though, in the moment of consuming them, they seem to be enlivening, stimulating, and pleasurable. These include such substances as alcohol, tobacco, flesh foods, and processed foods. You need not consume such substances for very long, nor need you consume them particularly to excess, in order to become aware of their toxifying effects. To use them at all will toxify and enervate you to a degree, depending on your metabolism and your state of health in general.[5]

Indeed, even the foods that are essentially sustaining and easily eliminated can also toxify and enervate you, if not taken in the right balance or if eaten to excess. Your ordinary functional life itself can toxify and enervate you. Sexual activity can toxify and enervate you. All of your ordinary involvements can wear you out and obstruct you—not only physically, but emotionally, mentally, psychically. You are the evidence of it. The entire society in which you live is the evidence of it!

People everywhere are commonly toxified and enervated by tobacco, alcohol, killed food, junk food, drugs—and bad company! Some just have a somewhat better ability to keep smiling, to keep laughing, longer than others. Yet, it is commonplace for people to die from toxic, enervated, and diseased conditions, and the cause of death is presumed to be some particular disease. However, the presumption of disease is just part of the "philosophy" that you are not loved to begin with, that you are cut off from what sustains, that you are mortal, and (therefore) that everything you do is tending to kill you.

Now, it is true that death is part of the cycle of life. At some point, the gross aspect of the body-mind is eliminated, like the unusable portion of food—literally eliminated, thrown off in the natural process, just like the blossoms of flowers. Flowers eliminate themselves. They obviously want to live—they made the gesture to begin with. Why do they not just go on living? No one needs to pick them—they die anyway. They do not die from sickness. They simply pass through a cycle of appearance, and then they disappear.

Similarly, the human being is structurally potentiated toward death, or the elimination of the gross part. Yet, death need not—and should not—be the result of toxicity and enervation. Such an end is simply a social consequence of ignorant, foolish habits and irresponsibility. One should die healthy, not from a long period of disease and suffering and wretchedness and senility or accidents and all the rest of the craziness that happens to a human being in this desert-world.

Basically, a human being should live quite a long life, of perhaps one hundred years or more. Perhaps you will experience the cycle of aging, but not as degraded deterioration and disease. You should be essentially full and happy—simply becoming very tired one day, and then dying. So it should be for you. Human beings are structurally disposed to die in just that fashion.

Yet, human beings, in general, habitually die (instead) from toxicity and enervation, as well as from the degradation of unlove and doubting and fear and anger and all the rest of the effects of being bad company to everything.

People become habituated to patterns of more or less perpetual indulgence in a toxifying and enervating diet, as well as to patterns of all the other negative habits of life. They do not bring such patterns to an end—and, therefore, they do not pass through the process of elimination and regeneration. Therefore, such people create a cycle of habits of unlove and degeneration. They inevitably fall into patterns of negative psychological states, obsessive sexual desires, confusion, psychological distress—yet, really, they are simply suffering overloaded intestines and a bad blood condition! They have forgotten the Law. They have forgotten that for which they should be responsible.

As My devotee, your entire life must be the process of reception and release, assimilation and elimination. Your entire life must take into account this simple procedure, at every level of functioning—relative to diet, relative to the emotional-sexual dimension of your being, relative to all your relations, relative to exercise and action, relative to breath and thought and meditation and all forms of growth. This simple process of reception-release reflects the structure of the body-mind as a whole and does not make allowance for choices in either the direction of self-exploitation or the direction of self-denial. Therefore, as My devotee, you are not obliged to adopt a "lifestyle" of strategic asceticism. Rather, you are obliged to be love, and to be Happy, and to be Sustained Absolutely—and to be (from the ordinary "point of view") "ascetic" only in the sense of adhering to the simple process of eliminating toxic accumulations and gradually transcending your degenerative habits.

3.

AVATAR ADI DA SAMRAJ: Throughout history, human beings have been looking for something to sustain them. Everything from Jesus of Galilee to Krishna to *Amanita muscaria*, the "sacred mushroom", is claimed to be the "Panacea", the "Sustainer", the "Thing" that rejuvenates, that keeps one forever alive and full. Because of the (false) metaphysical presumption of unlove, people are always seeking for the "Sustainer" outside themselves. All over the world, and throughout human time, cults have developed around magical something-or-others that represent food, the connection to what sustains. All holy rituals are about food. Most often, the rituals literally involve food: the sacrificing of food, the eating of food, "this is my body, this is my blood", the killing of calves, the taking of things from the holy place and absorbing their energies. In the only-by-Me Revealed and Given Way of Adidam, the Sacrament of Universal Sacrifice,[6] which all My devotees engage daily, may also tend to be used in this cultic fashion, if right devotional responsibility in relationship to Me is not presumed.

The search for the cultic "Sustainer" (or "Food"), the "Food Deity", the "Edible Master", is a futile search—yet, it occupies people all over the world. The root-impulse of every culture, every society, every religion, is to find the "Edible Deity", to come into mystical—and even direct physical—contact with That Which Sustains Perfectly. This entire search, and its imaginary fulfillment in cultic occasions— these "meals", including even the ordinary daily meal—are simply the product of human error, human suffering, human irresponsibility. It is true that one must be sustained. One must come into immediate Communion with That Which Is Absolute. However, the cultic ritual of coming into contact with the "Edible Deity", the great "Parent-Sustainer", is not true sustenance. That ritual is a form of delusion, a form of eating in the desert. It is plunder.

It may be said that the tradition of the so-called "Savior" that is found all over the world is a religious dimension of the search for the "Edible Deity". Yet, there are also cults all over the world that surround edible things—magical edible things, important edible secrets known only to a few. At the most elemental level, there are foods that are simply good for you, or herbs that will rejuvenate you, or herbs that will make you hallucinate and suddenly see something that is remarkable, something that intoxicates you and makes you feel happy. In the present time, many people are trying to identify various plants and other substances (from secret, far-off places all over the world) as the true "soma"[7]—which, when taken, completely rejuvenates you and makes you an immortal. The partaking of soma and the traditional taking of bread and wine are simply two versions of the same basic ritual. Many people are actively looking for the soma—just as people are actively looking for parent-like "saviors", or cultic "edible deities".

However, if you examine the entire argument that I have presented to you, perhaps you can understand that the true soma is not something you can eat. The true soma is the transformative internal secretion of the body-mind in its Prior (or Divinely Enlightened) State. In that State, the body-mind naturally secretes all the substances that rejuvenate it, enliven it, keep it psychically awakened and aware in the fullest possible sense.

Now you are toxic, enervated, your energy and attention are bound exclusively and strategically to certain functions—essentially, the gross functions of money, food, sex, and social egoity. You are in conflict. Your blood is impure. Your cells are full of toxic accumulations. You are socially disturbed and in mystery about everything altogether, waiting for something sustaining to appear on TV! Somebody—so you hope—is going to make an announcement on TV someday, about the ultimate, absolute, scientific, newsworthy discovery. The "Edible Deity" is going to appear there someday. Today's newscasters, if they live that long, may be privileged to announce it. Then millions of people will go and join that cult.

The cults of the "Edible Deity" are still appearing everywhere. People try to "eat" Me! People come to Me for the purpose of establishing a cult, to engage in a conventional and irresponsible association with Me as the "Edible Source" at the center. My true devotees—who are living in heart-Communion with Me, enjoying the advantage of right relationship to Me—are responsible, in daily practice, for the simple process, the Law, of their own structural being. Therefore, the functional body-mind of My true devotee continues to grow. It becomes purified and rejuvenated in the ordinary manner. And, from time to time, My devotees may fast and rejuvenate themselves.

However, the true soma is not eaten in the form of any objective meal. The soma is the substance that is <u>released</u> in the body when one lives the law of sacrifice. The soma is released in the most absolute Divine Enjoyment. It is the nectar of Amrita Nadi,[8] the Current of Immortal Bliss— "amrit" is the ancient word for the Divine Nectar. In some sense, this is a physiological process—the glands of the subtle structures of the body-mind[9] begin to secrete substances that are presently suppressed, because of the impure condition of the blood and the attenuated energy and attention of the being. These substances, secreted by the glands, rejuvenate and awaken the various psycho-physical centers.

The soma of the whole body is not accumulated in cultic fashion. In the Most Ultimate Realization of Truth, you are not simply sustained and made immortal in objective independence. Rather, you, as the apparently separate psycho-physical "self", are made a perfect sacrifice. You are made immortal not by accumulating benign things from without but by relinquishing the entire cycle of assimilation and elimination to Infinity. The body-mind becomes an offering thrown into the Eternal Fire of the Infinite Divine Self-Radiance. You become immortal by dying as the separate self—while alive.

The death of the elemental vehicle—toward which all living beings are naturally and ultimately disposed—is not a negative process. It is not the result of unlove, and it does not occur at the end of a degrading process of toxicity and enervation. As a human being, you are structurally disposed to be Awakened, whole bodily, through the built-in cycle of growth toward which your birth moves you. If you are My devotee, I Call you to live your human birth from the "point of view" of the heart, or of love. If you do so, then, most ultimately (by Means of My Avataric Divine Spiritual Grace), you come to the point where you spontaneously relinquish the entire body-mind to Infinity. That event is true ego-death, the true elimination of your independent, conditionally man-ifested, bodily, apparently separate existence. "You" dissolve in space and time—and the body is laid down in an appar-ently natural death at the appropriate time.

Death is where you are going, you see. From the egoic (or "Narcissistic") "point of view", death is a torment, the result of "sin" (or of "missing the mark", or unlawful action), unlove, toxicity, and enervation. It is a dreadful possibility. Consequently, everyone is trying to find the "Edible Deity"— in order to keep on living. Everyone seeks such a fake immortality. Yet, even structurally, everyone is disposed to die—just as the flowers cycle toward death with ease, and show no negative signs at all. In Truth, you are clarified, immortalized, glorified, by dying to the ego-"I".

And you return to the planes of conditionally manifested experience again and again—until you can be a sacrifice in every dimension. When you become that sacrifice in any plane, then you are moved beyond that dimension of expe-rience—which has become unnecessary to you because you have become a sacrifice there, not because you have turned away from it or wrenched yourself out of it through conven-tional Yogic or mystical activity, the inverting of attention and the going "up" and "away".

Through Most Perfect heart-Communion with Me (or That Which Sustains you), you are (most ultimately) Divinely Translated[10] into My Divine Self-Domain of "Brightness"[11]— Which Is Beyond even all the heavens, and Which has no archetype or symbol in your present mind and psyche.

Diet Is Not
the Key to Salvation

A Talk by
Avatar Adi Da Samraj

AVATAR ADI DA SAMRAJ: Diet is not the key to anything sublime. Diet is just food. Eating is vital (physical) activity. One cannot become absolutely healthy simply by manipulating the diet, because diet only addresses the body and not anything higher than the body in the range of functions. Diet does not deal with the more subtle levels of conscious awareness, the psychic being or the higher mental being. Because much of human existence is rooted in these subtle functions, not everything that is symptomatic in the vital (physical) life can be cured by the manipulation of vital-physical quantities such as food.

Therefore, do not seek the "perfect diet" in order to be "perfectly cured". There is an appropriate use of food—but, otherwise, diet does not deserve any attention whatsoever. My devotees are Called, by Me, to engage the fundamental practice of devotion to Me at every level of life. Thus, My devotees are Called, by Me, to adapt (simply, routinely, and happily) to the appropriate form of every life-function— without seeking "solutions", as if there were a "problem". If you live in devotional relationship with Me, then you do not need solutions!

Nevertheless, it does happen that, when a person who has been on a degenerative diet adapts to a healthful diet, his or her entire functional mind is changed. By means of fasting and right diet, all the mechanisms that feed the brain, that bring blood to the brain and transfer nerve-energy, are purified, intensified, and rejuvenated. Naturally, this process has a positive effect on the functional ability to use the mind in life, on the ability to think, to form concepts, to remember, to recall. All these functions are positively transformed in the process of purifying the physical life. In general, fasting and right diet certainly do tend to harmonize and clarify the psycho-physical life—but they do not transform the psycho-physical life absolutely.

If you simply regulate your life in accordance with physical laws, you will never completely transform or harmonize the psycho-physical life—because such complete transformation depends upon your application to laws that govern the subtle (emotional, mental, psychic, and mystical) functions of the body-mind, beyond the gross physical functions.

In general, food is necessary to varying degrees, depending upon one's present state of life, one's style of life, one's karmas, one's condition in the midst of life (entirely independent of what one does or does not do). If you are in conflict with yourself, you are always destroying the integrity of your functional life, and you depend upon things outside yourself to restore you. Therefore, you become very much dependent on sleep, food, and other substances that you can take into your body. You become very much dependent upon experiences from without, on promises from without, on sources of energy that are communicated from without.

However, simply because you observe that dependence in yourself does not necessarily mean that the opposite "ideal"—or a condition wherein you no longer eat, no longer sleep, no longer interact with anything that is apparently outside your functional personal presence in the world—is appropriate. Nearly everyone falls between these two extremes of dependence and independence, and you must inspect—and become responsible for—the play of your own dependence and independence. The rhythm of dependence and independence will change over time. It will even vary on any given day. For example, the pattern of sleep will change according to your present state of health, just as the degree of your energy will increase or vary over time, and the need for food and the entire effect of food on your life will vary over time.

It is true, however, that, if your general state of health is good, and if you keep active, exercise properly, and apply yourself to the recommended diet, you will need far less food—because the substances that you are consuming are alive and provide chemical elements that affect the vital (physical) system far more positively than the "junk" food that is commonly eaten by so many. You may also discover that you have less need for sleep at night.

Such questions as "Do human beings need food to survive?" or "Do human beings need sleep to survive?" have a certain experimental interest, but they are not fundamentally important. The relationship of the natural cycles to conscious awareness is significant. And it is in relation to conscious life—not, fundamentally, in relation to physical life in and of itself, or the need for survival—that all the life-disciplines (such as diet) have been Given, by Me, to My devotees. As a by-product of the appropriate management of diet, health and well-being improve, and these effects are certainly positive. The fundamental intention, however, is to produce the optimal condition for a conscious devotional life of sacrifice to the Divine Source-Condition of Reality, Truth, and Real (Acausal) God.

Nevertheless, people (including My devotees) can tend toward "lunch-righteousness". Right away, all kinds of goals of diet and physical life become very fascinating. For a period of several months, after I first Spoke about the discipline of diet and My devotees began to apply it every day, practically every time that someone came to Me, I was asked some question about diet. All anybody wanted to talk about was diet. The questions about diet were endless! People had become obsessed with diet—yet, it is only lunch!

Right diet is very simple—yet, as soon as a formal approach to a basic life-function is suggested, people begin to establish goals for the process. To My devotees at that time, everything about food and its use became fascinating. Suddenly everyone began to seek perfect health, longevity, immortality, and the Yogic body—through food. Yet there is no lunch—and there never has been a lunch, and there never will be a lunch—that can produce the Yogic body, or immortality, even extreme longevity or perfect health. There are a few basic principles relative to diet, and they are what they are. But, in and of itself, diet is not responsible for anyone's continued existence. A much larger circumstance than diet is responsible for your continued bodily existence, just as a greater Circumstance is responsible for your present bodily existence, and even your birth.

If there were a perfect goal that I could discover somehow and that seemed appropriate to Me, I would organize a system that would include every possible factor in life—because a perfect goal implies everything, and everything must be made to conform to it in one manner or another. However, there is no such goal. Your fetishistic preoccupation with goals is nonsense—the product, essentially, of suffering. Goals appeal to you because you are already suffering the sense of dilemma. Goals appeal to your sense of suffering, and only because of your present sense of suffering are you interested in attaining any goal at all.

In the early years of My Work with My devotees, before I determined that it was time for them to strictly observe the discipline of diet and other disciplines, people used to argue with Me about vegetarian diet and various other forms of diet—and I always argued against their persuasion. I smoked cigarettes in front of them, drank coffee deliberately, and talked about the entire strategy, the entire motivation, the entire false view of Spirituality that was their reason for being a vegetarian. I was not arguing against the vegetarian diet in and of itself, but against the strategic "program" that is connected with it. I have always Criticized the "program" that is your search—quite apart from whatever dietary regime you may be following.

Just as you must be free of self-indulgence and all of its goals, so also you must be equally free of the cult of discipline, the righteousness that appears whenever you self-consciously fulfill a discipline. Feeling self-conscious and modest while drinking a little mint tea with friends who are drinking coffee is so small, so narrow and tacky. It is the product of the cult of strategic self-discipline, in which there is no freedom, no fundamental humor, no real comprehension of the importance of daily events, but only foolish concerns for purity of diet when people are murdering one another with every movement of their minds. All such obsessive concern for diet is inappropriate. The appropriate approach to diet is simply a natural, functional awareness of what you eat.

Religious and Spiritual groups typically have some sort of cult of diet attached to them. And the more the members of any particular religious or Spiritual group adopt a "hard-line" stance (relative to such matters as diet), the more foolish, resistive, and alienated from the rest of the world they become. I do not expect My devotees to indulge themselves at all in the vulgar diet with which people in general are destroying themselves, but I do expect My devotees to have a humorous relationship to the world, to be present in the world without "making a fuss" about the fact that they engage certain practices and disciplines. In the midst of your application to right dietary practice, there are no grounds for righteousness or guilt or preoccupations. Work out your individual diet with intelligence, based on My detailed Instructions.

My interest is always to address the fundamental self-limiting activity of every human being. No matter what you are outwardly doing in any moment, the same self-obsessed one sits behind it. Therefore, I expect you to deal intelligently with your own functional life.

However, diet has nothing whatsoever to do with salvation—as you should know by now! The practice of diet is simply an ordinary discipline for intelligent people who are devoted to always present Communion with the Living Divine Reality, Truth, and Real (Acausal) God.

The Right and Optimum Diet

From "The ego-'I' is the Illusion of Relatedness",
An Essay by Adi Da Samraj
in *Santosha Adidam*

The grossest dimension of the body-mind is the physical body itself. It is associated with desire (or motive) and action based on desire. Therefore, the traditional path called "Karma Yoga" (or renunciation of the purposes and goals of the ego in the midst of bodily activity) was developed as a means to transcend bondage to bodily desire and activity (by surrendering the causes and the results of bodily action to the Divine—and this by converting all actions into forms of worship). Similarly, in the only-by-Me Revealed and Given Way of Adidam (Which is the One and Only by-Me-Revealed and by-Me-Given Way of the Heart), My devotee converts all of his or her actions into forms of ego-surrendering, ego-forgetting, and (more and more) ego-transcending Ruchira Avatara Bhakti Yoga.[12]

The gross body is, very simply, the food-body. The gross body (itself) depends on (and is made of) food. The quality and quantity of food largely (or very basically) determines the state and desire and action of the physical body and the sense-mind. If food-taking is intelligently minimized, and if the food selected is both pure and purifying, then the physical body (and even the entire emotional dimension of the being, and the total mind) passes through a spontaneous natural cycle that shows (progressive) signs of (first) purification, (then) rebalancing, and (finally) rejuvenation. Therefore, if food-taking is controlled, the physical body itself (including its desires and activities) becomes rather easily (or simply) controllable.

Because of this direct relationship between food-taking and the physical body, it is (in principle) very simple to restore the gross body to balance, health, and well-being. The basic treatment of any unhealthful condition of the gross body is a food-treatment (generally accompanied by rest from—or, otherwise, right and effective control of—all the enervating influences and effects of daily life). Therefore, primarily, it is through the food-discipline (accompanied by general self-discipline) that gross bodily purification, rebalancing, and rejuvenation are accomplished.

This "food-principle" is the fundamental physical basis of all physical healing. Some bodily conditions may require special healing treatments, but even such special approaches will be useful (in the fullest and long-term sense) only if accompanied by fundamental changes in diet (and simultaneous changes in one's habits of life). Therefore, always, the primary (and right) approach to physical health and physical well-being must be (first) to address (or examine) and (then) to treat (and to discipline) the gross body simply (or directly) as a food-process.

If the dietary (and the total) discipline of the body-mind is right, then (in the only-by-Me Revealed and Given Way of Adidam) attention can be more fully and freely (or less obstructedly, and more sensitively) Released to the practice of Ruchira Avatara Bhakti Yoga, and (thus, by Means of My Avatarically Self-Transmitted Divine Grace) to My Avataric Self-Revelation of the Acausal Divine Person and Self-Condition, and (Thus and Thereby) to My Direct (Avatarically Self-Transmitted) Divine Blessing (and, in the case of My Spiritually Active devotees, to My Avatarically Self-Transmitted Divine Blessing-Presence, or My Avatarically Self-Transmitted Divine Spirit-Current in—and, Ultimately, Prior to—the Circle and the Arrow of the body-mind[13]), and (Ultimately, and even from the beginning) to My Avatarically Given Divine Self-Revelation of Perfectly Subjective Being (Itself). If the dietary discipline of the body-mind and the Devotional feeling-discipline of attention (which discipline corresponds to the tradition of Bhakti Yoga[14]) are right, then all aspects of the gross (or frontal) personality[15] will be most easily (or most readily) economized and most easily (or most readily) conformed to the Devotional and (as My Avatarically Self-Transmitted Divine Spiritual Grace will have it) Spiritual Process of real—and (necessarily) whole bodily (or totally psycho-physically) surrendered—feeling-Communion with Me.

Therefore, the Yoga of right diet is a principal physical means (in the only-by-Me Revealed and Given Way of Adidam) whereby the body is utterly conformed to the Purpose of Most Perfect Realization of Real (Acausal) God, or Truth, or Reality. The ego would adapt the body-mind to purposes of worldly fulfillment and mere survival, but My devotee who rightly, truly, fully, and fully devotionally resorts to Me (and who, thus and thereby, understands egoity) no longer limits the body-mind to merely conventional and worldly purposes, but (rather) makes the body into a Yoga-body, through the exercise of Ruchira Avatara Bhakti Yoga (supported by all the disciplines of "conductivity" practice[16]).

In the Way of Adidam, the frontal Yoga (or right Devotional surrender of the frontal personality) takes place (or is begun) in the context of the fourth stage of life.[17] Therefore, it is a matter of the Devotional surrender of the gross body and the total frontal personality by means of ego-transcending Devotional (and, in due course, Spiritual) heart-Communion with Me.

The gross body depends on the various levels of the subtle body (and they, each in turn, depend on one another). There-fore, the gross body relates directly to the first level of the subtle body, which is the body of prana (or natural life-energy).

The natural ground of the gross bodily person is in the abdominal region, just below the umbilical scar—and, altogether, the natural ground of the gross bodily person includes all the functions within the total region extending from and through the solar plexus (to and through the general region of the navel) and all the abdominal functions below the navel. Therefore, once both the hearing of Me and the seeing of Me are established (and, indeed, as the entire listening, hearing, and seeing process[18] progressively becomes established), the practice of the Way of Adidam more and more fully becomes a matter of the true frontal Yoga of surrendering whole bodily (crown to toe) into My Avatarically Self-Revealed Divine Body of "Bright" Spirit-Force (thus and thereby Opening Upward to Me by exercising the feeling-level of the heart, Receiving Me, from above the head and mind, and allowing My Spirit-Fullness to Flow down to the bodily base).

Once the gross (or frontal) personality is under control (via a complex of disciplines associated with "money, food, and sex"—or life-relations, diet, and sexuality), and once My Avatarically Self-Transmitted Divine Spirit-Current is steadied in the frontal line from and via the central feeling-level (or heart chakra), then practice of the Way of Adidam has moved fully into the frontal (or descending) Yoga.

Among all the functional, practical, relational, and cultural disciplines that serve this frontal Yoga, the conservative discipline (or control) of diet is (elementally) the most basic—because dietary practice (which controls, or largely determines, the state of the food-body, or the state and general activity of the physical body) also determines the relative controllability of social, sexual, emotional, mental, and all other functional desires and activities.

If diet is controlled, the gross food-body is more easily controlled, and all the disciplines of the body-mind will be (to that degree) quickened in their effectiveness. Therefore, in the only-by-Me Revealed and Given Way of Adidam, right and optimum dietary discipline is a necessary basic aspect of practice (beginning at the student-beginner stage of the Way of Adidam[19]), and right and optimum dietary discipline (once it is thoroughly established, in the course of the student-beginner stage of the Way of Adidam) is a necessary basic characteristic of every (following) developmental stage of the Way of Adidam.

The right and optimum diet is (necessarily) a conservative diet. In right (or effective) practice of the Way of Adidam, dietary discipline fully serves the submission of personal energy and attention to the Great Process that becomes (Ultimately, by Means of My Avataric Divine Spiritual Grace) Most Perfect Divine Self-Realization. Therefore, the right and optimum diet must be intelligently moderated in its quantity and carefully selected in its quality, so that it will not burden the physical body or bind the mind (or attention) through food-desire and negative (or constipating, toxifying, and enervating) food-effects (and ingestion-effects in general), and so that (along with the necessary additional "consideration" and really effective transcending of aberrated, anxious, or even excessively private habits and patterns relative to food-taking and waste-elimination) it serves the yielding (or freeing) of functional human energy and attention to the great (and, necessarily, devotionally Me-recognizing and devotionally to-Me-responding) process (of self-surrender, self-forgetting, progressive self-observation, eventual most fundamental self-understanding, and, altogether, more and more effective self-transcendence, or real ego-transcendence) that is the necessary foundation of the only-by-Me Revealed and Given Way of Adidam. Consequently, right and optimum diet must (to the maximum degree that is both right and possible) be natural, fresh, whole, wholesome, balanced, balancing, pure (or non-toxic), and purifying—or, in the language of tradition, "sattvic".[20] And right and optimum diet must (to the maximum degree that is both right and possible) be limited to what is necessary and sufficient for bodily (and general psycho-physical) purification, balance, well-being, and appropriate service.

In the only-by-Me Revealed and Given Way of Adidam, right diet is whatever diet is (in any present moment) the "Minimum Optimum" diet for good health, well-being, and full practice of the Way of Adidam, in the case of the individual. Therefore, in the Way of Adidam, there is no absolute standard diet (applicable, in any and all moments, to all cases)—but, in the Way of Adidam, there is a basic dietary orientation (to which each individual must progressively adapt, to the maximum degree right and possible in his or her case), and that basic orientation is Given by Me as a dietary Rule and Guide for all formally acknowledged practitioners of the Way of Adidam. That basic orientation (or dietary Rule) is (to the maximum degree that is both right and possible, in the particular case of any individual practitioner of the Way of Adidam) to maximize the percentage of raw (and, altogether, "sattvic") foods, while including cooked (and, generally, "sattvic") foods only to the degree that (or during periods in an individual's life when) such cooked (and, generally, "sattvic") foods are (in one or another form) necessary for good health and well-being. (In the case of those who, whether consistently or for certain periods of time, require some cooked food in their diet, the fact that the cell walls are ruptured in cooked foods, thereby making calories more available in the process of assimilation, outweighs the otherwise definite health liabilities of cooked foods. The superior method of cooking most vegetables is wok cooking, because of the brief time required for cooking. However, the superior method of cooking such starchy vegetables as potatoes, yams, and winter squashes is steaming or baking.)

In the only-by-Me Revealed and Given Way of Adidam, the basic diet (to be—as a general, or daily, rule—formally expected of all student-beginners in the Way of Adidam, and of all practitioners at any stage of the Way of Adidam beyond that of student-beginner—unless, in any particular case, an individual is, rightly, medically advised to include a broader range of foods in his or her diet) is the diet that most fully and consistently meets all the requirements for right diet (or the "Minimum Optimum"—and, as a general daily rule, consistently "sattvic"—diet) I have Indicated. That diet (the healthful virtues of which have been fully experientially confirmed by Me, as well as by tradition, and by "modern" research and experimentation) is the (to the maximum degree that is both right and possible) vegetarian (or, more properly, fructo-vegetarian) diet—consisting maximally of raw (or uncooked, or unfired, and, thus, entirely living) foods.[21] That dietary discipline permits a range of possibilities, from an exclusively raw fructo-vegetarian (fruit-and-vegetable) diet to a maximally raw fructo-vegetarian (fruit-and-vegetable) diet (consisting of both raw and cooked foods in varying degrees). In either case, that basic (or "Minimum Optimum") diet is limited to fruits, seeds, nuts,[22] sprouts, greens, grasses, grains, legumes, and other vegetables. In the case of such a dietary discipline, foods are taken in both solid and liquid forms (except during fasts, or during any period in which an exclusively liquid fruit, or liquid vegetable, or liquid fruit-and-vegetable diet is preferred), and food is to be taken only in moderate amounts, using vitamins or other supplements only if (rightly) medically so advised.

During periods of intentional purification, systematic release, and generally reduced intake, the "Minimum Optimum" diet I have Described is usually restricted exclusively to raw foods (even in liquid form)—and, at other times (of constructive increase and general bodily development and maintenance), some intelligently measured amounts of cooked food may (as necessary) be taken. Nevertheless, the Basic Rule of this dietary design is that food should be (to the maximum degree possible and appropriate in the individual's case) restricted to raw substances, generally limited to the range of possibilities I have Described, and including cooked food only to the degree that some kind and amount of cooked food is found to be necessary for weight maintenance, bodily strength, balanced health (or general and healthful equanimity), and basic vitality and well-being. (The reason that the cooking, or firing, of foods is, in general, not optimal is that heat destroys the enzymes, heat-sensitive vitamins, and other heat-sensitive nutrients naturally present in raw foods, and it also changes the chemical structure of proteins and sugars in raw foods such that these proteins and sugars become less usable by—or even harmful to—the body.[23])

In order to understand and evaluate the "Minimum Optimum" ("sattvic", and maximally raw) dietary discipline (or disciplined dietary practice) Given by Me for application by all practitioners formally embracing the Way of Adidam, you should study the total (and progressive) "sattvic" dietary approach communicated in My Summaries of Instruction relative to dietary discipline.[24] Likewise, as a further aid to your understanding and evaluation of the by-Me-Given "Minimum Optimum" dietary discipline, you should (by means of a systematic, guided study of the traditional and "modern" literature I have Collected and Described for this purpose[25]) become familiar with the total tradition, including rightly-oriented "modern" research and experimentation, relative to "sattvic" (or pure and purifying, rebalancing, and rejuvenating) dietary discipline. Such study is a useful support to your embrace of the by-Me-Given "Minimum Optimum" dietary discipline. In your application to that discipline, I Call you to always intensively engage its progressive development—always artfully (and appropriately, or as necessary, and without abandoning the by-Me-Given "Minimum Optimum" dietary principles) taking into account such present-time factors as climate and season, the availability (and the quality) of locally grown food, the availability (and the quality) of food in general, the level of your physical (and mental, and emotional) purification, the state of your health in general, the degree and kind of your daily activity, and even all the factors associated with your age, your degree of vitality, your psycho-physical type,[26] and your developmental stage of practice in the Way of Adidam.[27]

And always practice the by-Me-Given dietary discipline with appropriate medical advice and supervision, so that the pace, the special requirements, and the results of your application of the by-Me-Given "Minimum Optimum" dietary discipline can be determined most efficiently and organized most effectively.

As a student-beginner in the Way of Adidam, begin (unless, correctly, medically advised otherwise) by embracing (and progressively developing and refining) a basic fructo-vegetarian (fruit-and-vegetable) diet, which diet should (in the general case) consist of both raw and cooked foods (and, if strictly necessary, some, generally small and occasional, amounts of milk and milk products), and develop (and refine) your basic dietary practice while you also develop and refine all the other basic (functional, practical, relational, and cultural) requirements for self-discipline in the only-by-Me Revealed and Given Way of Adidam.

Each and every practitioner of the only-by-Me Revealed and Given Way of Adidam is Called by Me (and is always to be formally expected) to constantly and intensively maintain the self-discipline of bodily purification, bodily rebalancing, and bodily rejuvenation (or bodily regeneration). As a basic means to quicken the effectiveness of your by-Me-Given (and formally expected) obligation to constantly and intensively maintain the self-discipline of bodily purification, bodily rebalancing, and bodily rejuvenation (or bodily regeneration), your dietary practice should also include right occasional and periodic fasting (unless you are otherwise rightly medically advised). Therefore, unless your bodily state (of <u>fully</u> achieved purification) and the purity of your daily food-intake do not (at any present moment) require it, your dietary practice should (if right medical advice permits) also (as necessary) include appropriate occasional (twenty-four-hour, or longer) and regular (extended) annual fasting. Such fasts should consist of the avoidance of all food intake—except for one or another (or, perhaps, a combination) of pure water, pure water with a small amount of lemon juice (or other citrus juice, or other fruit juice) added, pure water extracts of vegetables (otherwise known as "de la Torre" drinks[28]), raw (and, perhaps, diluted) fruit juices, raw (and, perhaps, diluted) vegetable juices, thin (or light) vegetable broths, and herb teas. Long fasts are to be engaged at least once per year (unless right medical advice prohibits such, or, otherwise, an exceptional state of bodily and dietary purity makes such, at any present moment, unnecessary)—and, to be effective, they should be continued for at least seven to ten days, and up to three or four weeks (or even longer). In addition, shorter or longer periods of exclusively raw diet (or, perhaps, of raw mono-diet) may also be engaged for the purpose of continuing the process of bodily purification during periods of time before and after fasting—but such temporary (rather than regular and constant) raw-diet exercises should be engaged only <u>in</u> <u>addition</u> to fasting, and not as an <u>alternative</u> to fasting (unless right medical advice suggests a period of raw diet as an alternative to fasting).

Refine (or simplify) your diet progressively, and, thus (but as directly and quickly as possible), pass through the necessary cycles of purification, rebalancing, and rejuvenation—until, in the course of student-beginner practice of the Way of Adidam, the discipline of "Minimum Optimum" diet (in the manner that has been demonstrated to be right and appropriate in your particular case—and with food taken always in minimum, but adequate, quantities) is stably achieved.

All those who would advance from the student-beginner stage to the intensive listening-hearing stage[29] of the Way of Adidam must (as a prerequisite) naturally exhibit basic psycho-physical equanimity, and they must (therefore) practice optimum dietary purity, simplicity, and moderation (in the manner I have herein Described). Once the transition is made from the student-beginner stage to the intensive listening-hearing stage of the Way of Adidam, the consistent practice of dietary purity, simplicity, and moderation must be continued (even in all the developmental stages beyond the intensive listening-hearing stage of the Way of Adidam), and such a practice (once established) will naturally tend to be continued (and, therefore, must be formally expected to continue), even in the context of the only-by-Me Revealed and Given seventh stage of life (in the Way of Adidam).

Any individuals (at the student-beginner stage of the Way of Adidam, or at any formally acknowledged developmental stage beyond the student-beginner stage of the Way of Adidam) who are medically (and correctly) advised to (either temporarily or regularly) include a broader range of foods in their diet, as their right form of the "Minimum Optimum" approach to diet—including (perhaps) a great percentage of cooked foods, and (perhaps) milk and milk products (even beyond the earliest phase of dietary adaptation), and (perhaps) also eggs, or (perhaps) even flesh food (whether fish, fowl, or animal),[30] and (perhaps) with therapeutic doses of vitamins and other food supplements as well, in addition to a basic diet of fruits, nuts, seeds, sprouts, greens, grains, legumes, and various other vegetables—may, of course, do so (under right medical supervision, and, as must be the case relative to even every matter of practice and discipline in the Way of Adidam, always with the formal agreement of the formal sacred cooperative cultural gathering of all formally acknowledged practitioners of the Way of Adidam[31])—but they should do so without self-indulgence, and strictly for health reasons, and only as a concession to necessity, and with constant sensitivity (and ego-transcending response) to the effects such foods produce in the body-mind, and on personal energy, and on attention. In many (or even most) cases, any such plan (if, rightly, medically required) would be related to the treatment either of some varieties of disease or of constitutional weakness that are (at least temporarily) not amenable to the optimum "sattvic" dietary approach. And no individual should (except in the case of a right, positive, and entirely justifiable health exception) be accepted for transition from the student-beginner stage to the intensive listening-hearing stage (or to any developmental stage of practice beyond it) who has not fully, consistently, and healthfully adapted to a maximally raw fructo-vegetarian diet, managed in real and right accordance with My herein Given Rule and principles. (And, in order to be accepted for transition from the student-beginner stage to the intensive listening-hearing stage, or, thereafter, in due course, to any developmental stage of practice beyond it, any individual for whom right, positive, and entirely justifiable health exceptions to the maximally raw fructo-vegetarian diet have been rightly and formally agreed upon, by appropriate representatives of the formal sacred cooperative cultural gathering of the Way of Adidam, must fully, consistently, and healthfully manage his or her dietary practice, in real and right accordance with My herein Given principles.)

All formally acknowledged practitioners of the Way of Adidam must, as a consistent and absolute rule (established even from the beginning of each individual's formal acceptance into the initially adapting, or novice, phase of student-beginner practice), entirely avoid (and are to be formally expected to, as a consistent and absolute rule, entirely avoid) all use (with the possible exception only of token and merely symbolic use, as may sometimes be required by custom for respectful and right participation in, necessarily rare, sacred, or entirely ceremonial and non-personal, social occasions[32]) of the more common (or commonly used) intoxicants (such as tobacco, alcohol, or kava)—because the casual (and also cumulative) effects of these substances are deluding, degenerative, and unhealthful.

All formally acknowledged practitioners of the Way of Adidam must, as a consistent and absolute rule (established even from the beginning of an individual's formal acceptance into the initially adapting, or novice, phase of student-beginner practice), entirely avoid (and are to be formally expected to, as a consistent and absolute rule, entirely avoid) all use of "soft" drugs (such as cannabis), all use of the traditional hallucinogenic drugs (such as peyote, mescaline, psilocybin, ayahuasca, and so on), all use of the hallucinogenic drugs that have a traditional social use in certain cultures (such as opium, and so on), all use of the so-called "recreational" (or even "hard") drugs (without any tradition of sacred or social use) that have been developed by means of chemical processes (such as heroin, cocaine, LSD, methamphetamines, and so on), all use of the so-called "recreational" (or even "hard") drugs originally developed for medical purposes (such as barbiturates and amphetamines), and (indeed) all use of any otherwise medically inappropriate drugs that may be discovered or developed at any point in human history—because the casual effects (and, in general, even the inherent characteristics) of "soft" drugs (such as cannabis), "recreational" drugs (of any kind), hallucinogenic drugs, "hard" drugs, and otherwise medically inappropriate drugs are (generally) extremely deluding, degenerative, and unhealthful.

Every practitioner formally embracing the Way of Adidam must always remember and actively (by right practice) affirm that the Way of Adidam is, even from the beginning, a self-purifying and ego-transcending Way of life. Therefore, from the beginning of the Way of Adidam, the consistent avoidance of toxic (or otherwise non-"sattvic") substances is the necessary (and formally to be expected) rule of practice—with only relatively rare (or infrequent, brief, and rightly occasional) exceptions to this rule being appropriate, and this (unless flesh foods are, rightly, medically recommended for health) in the case of foods made of the flesh (or any body parts) of "animals" (in which case, fish and poultry are the "preferred", or most "sattvic", of flesh foods[33]), and (unless unavoidably required for functional reasons) in the case of coffee[34] (whereas either black tea or oolong tea or green tea—all of which, and especially green tea, are generally regarded to have even medicinal, and generally non-toxic, or at least relatively and maximally non-toxic, properties[35]—may be taken, as an alternative to coffee, whenever, or however often, a caffeine-containing psycho-physical stimulant is rightly and truly required, for either functional or medicinal reasons), and (except for unavoidable necessity—and, otherwise, only with the possible exception of relatively rare occasions, when food is used in a liberally celebratory manner) in the case of non-"sattvic" foods such as "junk" food, foods made with refined sugar and/or refined flour, foods manufactured with additives, and so on.

My any devotee who persists in habits of gross physical self-indulgence (including dietary self-indulgence) is inevitably desensitized to Me—both devotionally and Spiritually. Therefore, such habits of gross physical self-indulgence undermine (and work against) the effectiveness of the sadhana (or Way of Divine Self-Realization) that I have Given to My devotees. This is the reason why refinement of the physical body via a diet that is conservative (or "Minimum Optimum"), and maximally raw, and (generally, unless right medical reasons indicate otherwise) fructo-vegetarian, and via a conservative (and truly "sattvic") approach to food-taking (and body-maintenance altogether), is necessary in the only-by-Me Revealed and Given Way of Adidam.

Any use of even the more common (or commonly used) intoxicants (such as tobacco, alcohol, or kava)—and (to an even greater degree) any use of "soft" drugs (such as cannabis)—temporarily suppresses psycho-physical (and heart-specific, and brain-specific, and nervous-system-specific) sensitivity to My Spiritual Transmission—after an initial period of gross intoxication, in which such sensitivity may, at the gross level, seem (to the temporarily intoxicated user) to increase. The perennial popular (or common) wisdom relative to the law and lesson of "fun" always applies. If you play—you must pay! If you dance—you must pay the piper! Even the executioner has his price! And the longer and hotter the dance, the more you must pay—whether now or later! And the longer you wait to pay your fees, the more the fees compound and increase!

Therefore, only by entirely avoiding all use (with the possible exception only of token and merely symbolic use, as may sometimes be required by custom for respectful and right participation in, necessarily rare, sacred, or entirely ceremonial and non-personal, social occasions) of even the more common (or commonly used) intoxicants (such as tobacco, alcohol, or kava), and by entirely avoiding all use (without any exceptions whatsoever) of "soft" drugs (such as cannabis), "recreational" drugs (of any kind), hallucinogenic drugs, "hard" drugs, and otherwise medically inappropriate drugs—and by restricting the use of non-"sattvic" (or otherwise toxic) dietary substances (in general) to the infrequent, brief, and rightly occasional exceptions that may be appropriately allowed—can My devotee establish toxin-free functional equanimity, and true and full sensitivity to My Spiritual Transmission, and the possibility of continuing and furthering the Devotional and Spiritual Process of Realizing Me. Because all of this is so (and not for any moralistic or puritanical or idealistic reasons), My every devotee—from the beginning of his or her practice as a formally acknowledged novice student-beginner (and always thereafter) in the Way of Adidam—must (except, in a token and symbolic manner, as may sometimes be required by custom, for respectful and right participation in, necessarily rare, sacred, or entirely ceremonial and non-personal, social occasions) entirely avoid any and all use of socially common intoxicants (such as tobacco, alcohol, or kava). And—from the beginning of his or her practice as a formally acknowledged novice student-beginner (and always thereafter) in the Way of Adidam—My every devotee must (without any exceptions whatsoever) entirely avoid any and all use of "soft" drugs (such as cannabis), "recreational" drugs (of any kind), hallucinogenic drugs, "hard" drugs, and otherwise medically inappropriate drugs.

The universal human (and ego-bound, and ego-binding) tendency to desensitize the body-mind to Me through indulgence in gross (or non-"sattvic") psycho-physical habits of any and every kind is the first and essential reason why (in the only-by-Me Revealed and Given Way of Adidam) there must be the right and consistent exercise of "sattvic" disciplines of the gross physical (and of the entire body-mind). Therefore, in the only-by-Me Revealed and Given Way of Adidam, the "sattvic" disciplining of gross (or non-"sattvic") psycho-physical habits in general, and of dietary self-indulgence in particular, is not a puritanical matter, or a moralistic matter— nor is it an idealistic matter. My devotees are not Called by Me to discipline the body-mind as a form of psycho-physical negativity (or body-denial), or as a form of utopian search for perfection in the context of conditionally manifested existence. Rather, in the only-by-Me Revealed and Given Way of Adidam, the "sattvic" disciplining of the body-mind (including the general, and right-principled, relinquishment of gross, or non-"sattvic", psycho-physical habits—and the consistent whole bodily, or total psycho-physical, and altogether right-principled, embrace of truly "sattvic" psychophysical disciplines) is simply a necessary and homely part of the realistic, and practical, and really and practically counter-egoic approach to Me, and to the Real Process of Devotional, and (in due course, as My Avatarically Self-Transmitted Divine Spiritual Grace will have it) Spiritual, relationship to Me—which relationship (formally, and fully accountably, embraced and practiced), and not any mere self-applied and ego-serving (or ego-improving, or even body-mind-improving) techniques, is (itself) the only-by-Me Revealed and Given Way of Adidam.

The total transition from conventional (or worldly) dietary practice to (an individually appropriate) practice of "Minimum Optimum" diet is a matter of a properly planned (and, as necessary, even medically supervised) transitional and progressive process of functional (and even mental and emotional) adaptation. Unless appropriate medical advice determines a different dietary accommodation, the progress of dietary adaptation should (as a general rule) proceed from basic fructo-vegetarian (or, if strictly necessary, lacto-fructo-vegetarian) dietary practice, and then to a maximally raw fructo-vegetarian (fruit-and-vegetable) dietary practice (generally, without milk or milk products). And, unless appropriate medical advice determines a different dietary accommodation, the total transition to a fructo-vegetarian (fruit-and-vegetable) diet that is consistently maximally raw must take place before the practice-transition beyond the student-beginner stage of the Way of Adidam can be formally approved.

As a general rule, the progressive process of adaptation to a fructo-vegetarian (fruit-and-vegetable) dietary practice that is consistently maximally raw may rightly take several months (or, in some, relatively rare, cases, even longer), with the actual transition-time determined by the previous habits, the strength of intention, and the general state of health of the individual. And, in <u>every</u> case, that achievement (or, otherwise, the achievement of right practice of any medically necessary variation on the "Minimum Optimum" diet), when it is right and real and true, is always (and necessarily) associated with profound and life-practice-converting discoveries about the body-mind-self—such that further advancement in the practice of the Way of Adidam is (thereby) given an extraordinarily positively transformed psycho-physical basis.

My Summary Instruction about the dietary discipline in the only-by-Me Revealed and Given Way of Adidam is (like all the Instruction Given by Me relative to the functional, practical, relational, and cultural disciplines of the Way of Adidam) the result of many years of examining all potential alternative orientations—as part of My own Avataric Ordeal of Divine Re-Awakening and My Avataric Self-Submission to Teach. Out of this process came My Summary Communication about the principles of the "Minimum Optimum" approach to dietary practice, as well as My Criticism of the dietary practice of the usual person, and even My Criticism of the false view (or misunderstanding) of diet as a so-called "Spiritual" practice.

I have used the term "lunch-righteousness" to describe the kind of mentality that seeks "salvation through diet". "Salvation through diet" is not part of the Way of Adidam I have Revealed and Given. Rather, My Instruction on right and optimum diet is a Teaching-Message from Me. It is a form of Dharma,[36] or right life. It is part of the foundation practice of self-discipline in the only-by-Me Revealed and Given Way of Adidam, to be practiced by My devotee in devotional recognition-response to Me. The dietary recommendation in the Way of Adidam is not a message about health (although health is certainly a result of right diet). Rather, the dietary recommendation in the Way of Adidam is a practice for My devotees. Therefore, the practice of right and optimum diet in the Way of Adidam is a devotional practice. It is a practical discipline assumed on the basis of devotion to Me.

This understanding of the dietary discipline in the only-by-Me Revealed and Given Way of the Heart (or Way of Adidam)—and, indeed, right understanding of all forms of functional, practical, relational, and cultural self-discipline in the Way of Adidam—tends to be obscured by the <u>search</u> for health and well-being. The lack of right understanding relative to practical self-discipline engenders all kinds of egoic misinterpretations relative to the practice of self-discipline. Such is not the Way of Adidam that I have Revealed and Given, and My devotees must be sensitive to the tendency to abandon right understanding of the by-Me-Given forms of self-discipline.

All aspects of the Way of Adidam—and, therefore, all aspects of the functional, practical, relational, and cultural disciplines of the Way of Adidam—are forms of My Avatarically Given Divine Wisdom-Teaching. All aspects of the Way of Adidam have to do with the relationship to Me and the process of the sadhana of devotion to Me. Every form of My practical Instruction on self-discipline is a <u>Teaching-Argument</u>, and not merely a communication of the "subject matter", in and of itself. Therefore, every presentation of My Avataric Divine Instruction involves My Criticism of egoity and of particular aspects of what people tend (egoically) to do in that area of life. Furthermore, every presentation of My Avataric Divine Instruction relative to any aspect of the forms of self-discipline in the Way of Adidam carries a Criticism of the particular stage of life that can be said to be the dominant orientation associated with each form of self-discipline.

For instance, the discipline of right and optimum diet (generally speaking) is applied in the context of the first three stages of life, and, therefore, in the context of egoity in the terms of the first three stages of life. My Wisdom-Teaching about diet is, first of all, founded in devotion to Me, and, additionally, Presents the principle of right and optimum diet through the mode of Argument in relation to other possibilities that might arise in the egoic approach to diet in the context of the first three stages of life.

My Wisdom-Teaching about the functional, practical, relational, and cultural disciplines of the Way of Adidam is not merely a message about health. Obviously, My practical Instruction to My devotees relates to matters of health, but the improvement of one's health is not the principal purpose of the by-Me-Given forms of self-discipline. Likewise, My Avataric Divine Wisdom-Teaching cannot be reduced to an Address to egoity merely in the mode of the first three stages of life, nor to an Address to fantasies about more advanced stages of life—nor is My Wisdom-Teaching to be made subordinate to messages coming from the existing religious and Spiritual traditions.

Much of the popular literature on diet that purports to relate to Spiritual practice, or sadhana—even much of the popular communications about vegetarian diet and raw diet altogether—tends to be associated with lunch-righteousness, faddism, and hype, and even a kind of "messianic" approach to communicating about diet by people who are (generally speaking) merely deluded by their own energies.

My Communication about diet is "bland" by comparison. It is not hyped. It is not offering "glorious salvation" by means of lunch. The bare facts of the dietary principles in the Way of Adidam are not, in and of themselves, particularly interesting, or made appealing by means of fascinating gimmicks. The principles of the right and optimum (or "sattvic") dietary approach I have Given are a very direct address to real matters of practical living—including, principally, many forms of My Criticism of egoity in the mode of self-indulgence and the misuse of diet as a form of consolation, as well as My Criticisms of faddism, or the search for salvation through diet.

My Communication about diet is a reasonable and flexible approach that must be practiced with great intelligence and as part of a process of real self-observation, accountability within the cooperative cultural gathering of My devotees, and right medical guidance (even in terms of modifying the diet based on particular conditions, both personal and environmental). My Communication about right and optimum diet is an offering of specific principles that can be applied in every individual case.

Those who are vulnerable to fascination with diet and "lunch gurus" may tend to bring such notions to the study of My Instruction and try to find the same fascination in My Communications about right diet. Others, who are self-indulgent, resist the maintaining of self-discipline altogether. Both these false approaches to sadhana—the "messianic" (or "lunch-righteous") and the self-indulgent—are (and must be) Criticized by Me. My Instruction relative to right diet Addresses the tendencies toward exaggeration—either exaggeration via self-indulgence or exaggeration via the absurdity of "messianic lunchism" (or the illusion that diet somehow leads to Divine Realization).

Right diet does not (and cannot) cause Divine Realization. In fact, right diet (in and of itself) has nothing to do with Divine Realization (Itself). Therefore, in the only-by-Me Revealed and Given Way of Adidam, right diet is simply and only a practical discipline.

My Instruction about right diet consists of general principles—and My Instruction about right diet also includes exceptions to those general principles, for people with particular health problems. The principles of the practice of diet

Communicated by Me are a basis for an intelligent approach to dietary practice. A characteristic of the dietary practice in the Way of Adidam is that it is without extremes. It is simply an intelligent approach to the matter. It is not a diet for seekers.

In making an intelligent approach to dietary practice, it is critically important that you rightly manage the transition from a conventional (or worldly) diet to the form of the "Minimum Optimum" diet that is right and appropriate in your particular case—otherwise, your unpreparedness will likely cause you to feel that the by-Me-Given dietary principles do not work in your case.

The "Minimum Optimum" (or "sattvic") dietary approach is part of My Instruction, and it is simply the form of dietary practice that naturally fits within the total structure of right principles I have Communicated. Therefore, My dietary Instruction is not based in any grandiose claims about raw diet (in and of itself), as if a diet of raw food is some kind of "messianic" solution to the problems of humanity.

One's diet is a straightforward, practical matter—and the practice of <u>right</u> diet is likewise straightforward. One must learn about diet, of course, but its application in practice should be so straightforward, from day to day, that the total life of right practice is not burdened with exaggerated attention to the physical dimension of the being.

People who are intensely involved in dietary seeking are constantly occupied with their search. Such people become deluded by their own energies and fascinations, and they exaggerate the importance of diet—thinking, in fact, that diet has something to do with Spiritual consciousness. Diet, in and of itself, has <u>nothing</u> to do with either Spirituality Itself or Consciousness Itself. Food-taking is simply a biological practice. Therefore, the effective taking of food has to do with matters of biology and the principles of the living system and its reactions.

The practice of right diet is a bodily discipline, not a Spiritual discipline. The practice of right diet originates (and, essentially, belongs) in the context of the first three stages of life—or the physical platform on which all of psycho-physically activated sadhana is done. The practice of right diet does not itself extend into Spirituality. Indeed, I Criticize <u>all</u> notions that have to do with physical (or psycho-physical, or conditional) seeking for some ultimate state—including a Spiritual state, or extreme longevity, and so on.

Each and all of My Instructions relative to the functional, practical, relational, and cultural disciplines of the only-by-Me Revealed and Given Way of Adidam carry with them a Critical Address to <u>five</u> key points: egoity, seeking, the "yes"/"no" extremes on either side of the basic requirements of sadhana, stages-of-life prejudices (or any and all attachments to a particular developmental stage of life, and, also, to the resulting illusions), and Great Tradition attachments (or even any and all uninspected presumptions, of any kind). Each of those five key points is basic to My Instruction. Everyone has an orientation or a tendency in some direction or other that relates to these five key points. Therefore, My Address to right diet—and the address made to the dietary practice of My devotees by designated representatives of the cooperative cultural gathering of My devotees—must speak not only to the subject of a particular functional, practical, relational, or cultural form of discipline, but must make reference to these five key points. Every form of My Instruction is an Argument that Addresses the egoic tendencies in people. This Address should inspire people and help them to correct themselves in their life-practice. And such understanding of My Instruction clearly identifies the uniqueness of the Way of Adidam as My Avataric Divine Revelation.

Basic Practical Advice

An Essay by
Avatar Adi Da Samraj

Constantly cultivate those conditions of existence that permit or tend to be associated with the native state of the human being. The native state of the human being is equanimity, or the naturally radiant psycho-physical condition that is prior to any form of self-contraction.

Such practice is, ultimately, quite complex (and even technical) in its details, but it may also be summarized in the form of basic practical advice:

Conserve diet.

Conserve sex.

React less.

Think less.

Talk less.

Surrender more.

Relax more.

Trust more.

Love more.

Serve more.

Meditate more, and Really.

Create, choose, and value those environmental, social, and intimate circumstances that are compatible with the native state of human being.

As My devotee, you must turn to Me moment to moment, and (on the basis of such turning to Me) make the practical basics of the Way of Adidam your life-practice, and (thereby) develop more and more free energy and attention—free of obsessive, unbalanced, and over-stimulated involvement with the conventional, superficial, and apparently problematic conditions of existence.

Thus, over time, you will, in your moment to moment practice of turning to Me, Awaken more and more to My Avataric Divine Spirit-Presence—and, most ultimately, Awaken (by Means of My Avataric Divine Spiritual Grace) to the only-by-Me Revealed and Given seventh stage of life.

Key Dietary Principles from the Wisdom-Teaching of the Avataric Great Sage, Adi Da Samraj

by Charles Seage, MD

No "Lunch-Righteousness"

One of the most precious, interesting, and "radical" principles that Avatar Adi Da has Given relative to diet in the Way of Adidam is that of not indulging in what He calls "lunch-righteousness". Lunch-righteousness is the tendency to perceive diet as something that (in and of itself) has moral and Spiritual significance. As He has stated in the Talk "Diet Is Not the Key to Salvation" in this book, diet is a simple and straightforward matter. Right diet does not guarantee perfect health, nor does it guarantee Ultimate Spiritual Realization. The purpose of right diet is simply to enable the body to sustain itself physically, without building up toxic accumulations that would obstruct one's growth in the Spiritual process. Thus, right diet is not about the search for perfection, but (rather) is something ordinary, done simply to support the body. For devotees of Avatar Adi Da Samraj, right diet is primarily a devotional practice, engaged in the disposition of surrender to the Divine Source-Condition and in relationship to Adi Da Samraj as Divine Heart-Master. Understanding this principle is key to being able to correctly apply the other dietary principles Adi Da Samraj has Given.

The Basic Diet:
Maximally Raw, "Minimum-Optimum"

Right diet necessarily promotes equanimity. Right diet does not burden the body with toxic substances. Thus, a right dietary regime is not overly stimulating, nor does it cause the body-mind to be weak and unable to be present in life with energy. Right diet is balanced.

To achieve this type of diet, most people will find that what they eat should be maximally raw. And what is maximally raw? In our experience as devotees of Adi Da Samraj, we have found that it means 100% raw for a great majority of people. Certain conditions, of course, will require exceptions to the all-raw diet—such as the inability to maintain one's weight in a healthy range or certain illnesses or health conditions that require a different dietary approach. Thus, there are individual variations, but there are many more people who can eat a 100%-raw diet than might be expected. In any individual case, maximally raw could mean 100% raw, or it could mean something less than 100%, as absolutely required. In the general case (where there are no health conditions that require a certain percentage of cooked food), 100% raw is optimal, because the all-raw diet is the most nourishing and simultaneously the most purifying.

As Adi Da Samraj has indicated, the diet of each of His devotees must be individually determined—within the range of possibilities He describes—such that the foods a person eats are completely compatible with (and supportive of) the particular body-mind of the individual. That is how one works it out—by finding what works and what does not work, through intelligent experimentation (in consultation, as necessary, with a qualified medical professional).

Another principal aspect of right diet is "systematic undereating". This simple "rule" is one of the key health principles that must be incorporated into one's dietary practice, in order to avoid chronic health problems and toxicity. Stated simply, it means eating only what is necessary, and not to the point of feeling completely full. By tendency, we eat to feel full, because we are afraid of not getting enough sustenance—as Adi Da Samraj says in His Talk "Renouncing the Search for the Edible Deity" in this book.

The Raw Diet Is a Whole-Foods Diet, Not a "Cuisine"

The maximally raw, "minimum-optimum" diet is a whole-foods diet. The food should be as close as possible to its natural state—optimally, grown in your local area (or even in your own garden), and prepared by you in a simple yet wholesome and pleasing way. One should eat only a few different foods at each meal—not a conglomerate of everything you can find in the kitchen.

Thus, the raw-foods diet is not intended to be a "cuisine". Mimicking the appearance and taste of cooked foods only reinforces old habits of using food as a form of consolation. Of course, on special occasions, a more elaborate raw meal might be prepared as a celebratory feast.

Refinements to the Diet: Cycles and Rhythms

There is an ongoing refinement of the diet which includes cycles of purification and nourishment. A person needs to vary the diet according to how the body feels. Even on the maximally raw diet, one will discover that, after a time, the body comes to the point of not feeling as it should. This is a sign that it is time to eat a more purifying diet for a while, until the body is again ready for more nourishment. The body gives signals to which you must be sensitive. Therefore, you do not merely maintain a single uniform diet as a "formula", but you adjust and refine the diet according to the cycles that the body is experiencing. A period of purification could be engaged in the form of a fast—or, otherwise, simply by lightening the diet somewhat. For example, one may eat only fruit for a time. By always remaining aware of the state of the body, a person can support the body's involvement in what Avatar Adi Da calls the "three phases of healing": purification, balancing, and rejuvenation. Purification rids the body of toxicity (which is caused by a failure to eliminate psycho-physical waste). Balancing corrects any imbalance between the two halves of the autonomic nervous system (sympathetic and parasympathetic). And rejuvenation overcomes the enervation that is the loss of nerve-force and of the energizing chemistry of the endocrine system. The body-mind constantly shifts through the cycle of three phases, never staying in one phase. Dietary variations and changes are important to the three phases, along with other healing exercises.

Adi Da Samraj says that it is important for the body to enjoy the foods it is taking in. Thus, the body's response to different foods is a sign to which one must remain sensitive. It is not a matter of attempting to mentally determine what foods one should eat, nor is it a matter of preferring a certain style of "cuisine". The foods one eats should look good to the eye, taste good to the tongue, and feel good in the body—in a simple and direct manner.

Another matter of dietary sensitivity is discovering the appropriate upper and lower limits of your weight. By feeling the cycles (or rhythms) of nourishment and purification that the body goes through, and adapting the diet to these rhythms, one will come to know the highest weight at which one still feels good in the body and the lowest weight at which one still feels good in the body. Remaining sensitive to these weight-limits, and keeping the body-weight within that range, is another aspect of the dietary practice that Adi Da Samraj recommends.

The "Systems" Approach to Healing

Fasting and raw diet are extremely important principles for healing—especially in Avatar Adi Da's "systems" approach to health and healing. The usual approach to healing is analytical and objective: to seek for causes of ill health via tests, and so forth, and to treat the ailment "from the outside in". One takes substances into the body from outside, based on forms of objective analysis. But Avatar Adi Da's Wisdom, while not abandoning the positive and necessary aspects of this analytical approach, uses the "answers" that lie in the body itself. Many times the objective, purely scientific approach reveals nothing. However, Adi Da Samraj says that the body itself knows what is wrong—without being able to name the problem—and the body can generally do something about it, by undoing the causes of the problem at their root. He describes this as dealing with health problems "from the inside out".

How does one accomplish this? To a large extent, this can occur simply through the principles of fasting and maximally raw diet. After a period of fasting, many chronic health conditions either disappear altogether or are permanently improved to a significant degree, if one adopts a maximally raw diet, which constantly purifies the body and thus does not allow toxicity, imbalance, and enervation to establish themselves again.

Charles Seage, MD, received his medical degree from the State University of New York at Buffalo in 1969, and subsequently specialized in internal medicine. In 1978, Charles became a devotee of Adi Da Samraj. Charles presently lives at Adi Da Samrajashram (the Hermitage Ashram of Adi Da Samraj in Fiji) where he continues to practice medicine, on the basis of Adi Da's "radical" approach to healing, and to serve as Adi Da's personal physician (a service he has performed for over 20 years).

Notes to the Text of
The Yoga of Right Diet

Renouncing the Search for the Edible Deity

1. In one of His earliest Discourses to practitioners of the Way of Adidam, Avatar Adi Da used the phrase "vital shock" to describe the primal recoil of every individual from the experience of being born—and, throughout the course of egoic life, from the vulnerable condition of bodily existence and of relationship itself. (See "Vital Shock" in *My "Bright" Word*.)

2. In Avatar Adi Da's Teaching-Revelation, "Narcissus" is a key symbol of the un-Enlightened individual as a self-obsessed seeker, enamored of his or her own self-image and egoic self-consciousness.

> *He is the ancient one visible in the Greek myth, who was the universally adored child of the gods, who rejected the loved-one and every form of love and relationship, and who was finally condemned to the contemplation of his own image—until, as a result of his own act and obstinacy, he suffered the fate of eternal separateness and died in infinite solitude.*
>
> —Avatar Adi Da Samraj, *The Knee Of Listening*

Avatar Adi Da uses the adjective "Narcissistic" in the sense of "relating to the activity of self-contraction", rather than in any more conventional meaning (particularly those meanings associated with the discipline of psychology).

3. The fundamental presumption (and activity) of separation.

4. The gross dimension is one of the three fundamental dimensions of conditional existence—succinctly defined by Avatar Adi Da as "outer" (gross), "inner" (subtle), and "root" (causal). As manifested in the human being, the gross dimension is the physical body, the subtle dimension includes the etheric/emotional, mental, and observing/discriminating functions, and the causal dimension is the root of attention (or the sense of existing as a separate "I").

69

5. Note that Avatar Adi Da does indicate that, from among this list of foods to avoid, flesh foods (or "killed food") may be (rightly) medically advised in some cases. (See pp. 47–48.)

6. This is Avatar Adi Da's description of the simple "ceremony" of the exchange of gifts between Him and His devotee. The devotee offers the gift of selfless devotion to Avatar Adi Da—represented by a tangible offering—and He, in return, Gives His Avataric Divine Blessing.

7. "Soma" is a word used in ancient and traditional Indian society to describe a plant (or intoxicating juice) that was used in religious ceremonies. The exact plant or substance is not known, though a number of psycho-active mushrooms and seeds have been proposed. The term was also prominently used to describe an "opiate for the masses" in Aldous Huxley's novel *Brave New World*.

8. Amrita Nadi is Sanskrit for "Channel (or Current, or Nerve) of Ambrosia (or Immortal Nectar)". Amrita Nadi is the ultimate "organ", or root-structure, of the body-mind, Realized as such (in Its "Regenerated" form) in the seventh stage of life in the Way of Adidam.

9. See note 4.

10. This is a reference to what Avatar Adi Da Samraj has Revealed to be the final phase of the demonstration of the Most Perfect (or "seventh stage") Awakening. In the Great Event of Divine Translation, body, mind, and world are no longer noticed—not because one has withdrawn or dissociated from conditionally manifested phenomena, but because the Self-Abiding Divine Self-Recognition of all arising phenomena as modifications of the Divine Self-Condition has become so intense that the "Bright" Divine Conscious Light now Outshines all such phenomena.

11. Avatar Adi Da affirms that there is a Divine Self-Domain that is the Perfectly Subjective Condition of the conditional worlds. It is not "elsewhere", not an objective "place" (like a subtle "heaven" or mythical "paradise"), but It is the Divine Source-Condition of every conditionally manifested being and thing—and It is not other than Avatar Adi Da Himself.

The Right and Optimum Diet

12. Ruchira Avatara Bhakti Yoga is the principal Gift, Calling, and Discipline offered by Avatar Adi Da Samraj to His devotees.

The phrase "Ruchira Avatara Bhakti Yoga" is itself a summary of the Way of Adidam. "Bhakti", in Sanskrit, is "love, adoration, or devotion", while "Yoga" is "God-Realizing discipline" (or "practice"). "Ruchira Avatara Bhakti Yoga" is, thus, "the practice of devotion to the Ruchira Avatar, Adi Da Samraj".

The practice of Ruchira Avatara Bhakti Yoga is the process of turning the four principal faculties (body, emotion, mind, and breath) to Avatar Adi Da (in and <u>as</u> His Avatarically-Born bodily human Divine Form) in every moment and under all circumstances.

13. The Circle (which Adi Da Samraj sometimes refers to in this text as a "Circuit") is a primary pathway of natural life-energy and the Divine Spirit-Energy in the body-mind. It is composed of two arcs: the descending Current, which flows through the frontal line—down the front of the body, from the crown of the head to the bodily base—and which corresponds to the gross dimension of the body-mind; and the ascending Current, which flows through the spinal line—up the back of the body, from the bodily base to the crown of the head—and which corresponds to the subtle dimension of the body-mind.

Avatar Adi Da describes the Arrow as "The breathless and Moveless, but Upwardly Polarized, Central Axis . . . Of the Cosmically-Patterned body-mind", which can be felt in deepening meditation.

14. Traditional Hindu devotional Yoga, in relationship to a deity or a Spiritual Realizer.

15. The "frontal personality" is a reference to the aspect of the human being that is focused in the energy-pathway in the human structure (extending from the crown of the head to the bodily base) through which both the natural life-energy and the Divine Spirit-Energy flow downward (or in a descending direction). The frontal personality comprises the ordinary daily functions of body, emotion, and mind.

16. Avatar Adi Da's technical term for participation in and responsibility for the movement of natural bodily energies (and, when one is Spiritually Awakened by Him, for the movement of His Divine Spirit-Current of Love-Bliss in Its natural course of association with the body-mind), via intentional exercises of feeling, relaxing, and breathing.

17. Avatar Adi Da Samraj describes the experiences and Realizations of humankind in terms of seven stages of life. This schema is one of Avatar Adi Da's unique Gifts to humanity—His precise "mapping" of the potential developmental course of human experience as it unfolds through the gross, subtle, and causal dimensions of the being. He describes this course in terms of six stages of life—which account for, and correspond to, all possible orientations to religion and culture that have arisen in human history. His own Avataric Revelation—the Realization of the "Bright", Prior to all experience—is the seventh stage of life. Understanding this structure of seven stages illuminates the unique nature of Avatar Adi Da's "Sadhana Years" (and of the Spiritual process in His Company).

The first three (or foundation) stages of life constitute the ordinary course of human adaptation—characterized (respectively) by bodily, emotional, and mental growth. Each of the first three stages of life takes approximately seven years to be established. Every individual who lives to an adult age inevitably adapts (although, generally speaking, only partially) to the first three stages of life. In the general case, this is where the developmental process stops—at the gross level of adaptation. Religions based fundamentally on beliefs and moral codes (without direct experience of the dimensions beyond the material world) belong to this foundation level of human development.

The fourth stage of life is characterized by a deep impulse to Communion with the Divine. It is in the context of the fourth stage of life (when one is no longer wedded to the purposes of the first three stages of life) that the true Spiritual process can begin. In the history of the Great Tradition, those involved in the process of the fourth stage of life have characteristically felt the Divine to be a great "Other", in Whom they aspired to become absorbed, through devotional love and service. However, in the Way of Adidam, the presumption that the Divine is "Other" is transcended from the beginning.

In the Way of Adidam, the process of the first three stages of life is lived on the basis of the devotional heart-impulse that is otherwise characteristic of the fourth stage of life. No matter what the age of the individual who comes to Avatar Adi Da, there will generally be signs of failed adaptation to the first three stages of life. But the practice is not a matter of attempting to overcome such failed adaptation through one's own (inevitably egoic) effort or struggle. Rather, the practice is to turn the faculties of the body-mind to Avatar Adi Da in devotional surrender. In that manner, the virtue of the fourth stage of life—the devotional heart-impulse to Commune with the Divine—is specifically animated from the beginning, in living response to Avatar Adi Da. Thus, whatever must be done to righten the first three stages of life occurs in the devotional context of heart-Communion with Him.

Avatar Adi Da has Revealed that the true Spiritual process, beginning in the fully-established (or "basic") context of the fourth stage of life, involves two great dimensions—which He calls the "vertical" and the "horizontal".

The descending aspect of the vertical process characterizes the fourth stage of life, while the ascending aspect characterizes the fifth stage of life. As it has been known in the history of the "Great Tradition" of relogous and Spiritual Instruction, the fifth-stage process is the ascent toward absorption into the Divine Matrix of Light Infinitely Above, thereby (ultimately) Realizing the Divine as Light (or Energy) Itself. (Although this Realization is a true "taste" of the Divine Self-Condition, It is achieved by means of the conditional effort of ascent—and, therefore, the Realization Itself is also conditional, or non-permanent.) The fifth stage of life is the ultimate process associated with the subtle dimension of existence.

The horizontal process characterizes the sixth stage of life. As it has been known in the history of the Great Tradition, the sixth stage process is the exclusion of all awareness of the "outside" world (in both its gross and subtle dimensions), by "secluding" oneself within the heart—in order to rest in the Divine Self, Realized (ultimately) as Consciousness Itself. (Like the ultimate Realization associated with the fifth stage of life, the sixth stage Realization is also a true "taste" of the Divine Self-Condition.

However, It is also achieved by conditional means—the conditional effort of exclusion—and, therefore, the Realization Itself is also conditional, or non-permanent.) The sixth stage of life is the process associated with the causal dimension of existence.

As Avatar Adi Da has pointed out, even though the fifth stage and sixth stage processes are, in fact, stages in the single process that culminates in Most Perfect Divine Enlightenment (or the seventh stage Realization uniquely Given by Him), the typical traditional view has been that the two processes are <u>alternative</u> approaches to Spiritual Realization. Indeed, these approaches (of either going "Up" or going "Deep") have usually been regarded to be incompatible with each other.

The "Perfect Practice" of the Way of Adidam encompasses <u>both</u> the vertical process (otherwise characteristically associated with the fifth stage of life) <u>and</u> the horizontal process (otherwise characteristically associated with the sixth stage of life). Thus, in the Way of Adidam, there is no "preference" exercised in favor of either the "Upward" process or the "Inward" process—either the Realization of the Divine as Light Itself or the Realization of the Divine as Consciousness Itself. In the Way of Adidam, both the ultimate "Upward" Realization and the ultimate "Inward" Realization are Freely Given by Avatar Adi Da to the rightly prepared and rightly practicing devotee. No effort—either of ascent or of exclusion—is required. And, in fact, all such effort must be inspected, understood, and transcended.

This unique and unprecedented orientation to the developmental processes of the fifth and the sixth stages of life is made possible by the full reception of Avatar Adi Da's Gift of Divine Spiritual Transmission. When the devotee (in the context of the fourth stage of life in the Way of Adidam) is fully open to Avatar Adi Da's Divine Spiritual Transmission, His Divine Spiritual Descent of what He calls "the 'Thumbs'" takes over the body-mind, showing specific Yogic signs. In this "Samadhi of the 'Thumbs'", there is a profound turnabout in one's awareness of Him. While still always turning to Him devotionally in His bodily (human) Divine Form, one begins to recognize Him, Spiritually, as Consciousness Itself—the Root-Position of existence, Prior to all that is arising in body, mind, and world. This recognition is Spiritually established—and it is the basis for making the transition to the "Perfect Practice" of the Way of Adidam. It is a profound shift, away from identification with the body-mind. From this point on, Avatar Adi Da's Revelation of His own Condition of Consciousness Itself becomes the Position in which one Stands, and from That Position the phenomena associated with both the fifth stage of life and the sixth stage of life will arise. In the "Perfect Practice", one is no longer practicing from the "point of view" of the body-mind and its faculties. Now, devotional turning to Him (or Ruchira Avatara Bhakti Yoga) takes the form of simply "choosing" to Stand in His Position (rather than the ego-position)—inspecting and feeling beyond the root-tendency to contract and create the self-identity called "I".

The seventh stage of life, or the Realization of Avatar Adi Da's own "Bright" Divine Condition, transcends the entire course of human potential. In the seventh stage of life, the impulse to Realize the Divine (as Light) by going "Up" and the impulse to Realize the Divine (as Consciousness) by going "Deep" are (by Avatar Adi Da's Divine Spiritual Grace) simultaneously fulfilled. In that fulfillment, Avatar Adi Da Samraj Himself is most perfectly Realized. He is Realized as the "Bright", the Single Divine Unity of Consciousness and Energy—or Conscious Light Itself. This unique Realization, or Divine Enlightenment—first Realized by Avatar Adi Da Himself, in the Great Event of His Divine Re-Awakening—wipes away every trace of dissociation from the body-mind and the world. There is no impulse to seek or to avoid any experience. Rather, everything that arises is Divinely Self-Recognized to be merely a modification of the Conscious Light of Reality Itself.

The seventh stage Realization is absolutely Unconditional. It does not depend on any form of effort by the individual. Rather, It is a Divine Gift, Given by Avatar Adi Da to the devotee who has utterly surrendered all egoity to Him. Therefore, the seventh stage Realization is permanent.

Altogether, the Way of Adidam is not about dwelling in (or seeking to either attain or avoid) any of the potential experiences of the first six stages of life. The Way of Adidam is about transcending the entire structure of the human being and of the conditional reality—gross, subtle, and causal. Therefore, the Way of Adidam transcends both the urge to "have" experiences and the urge to "exclude" experience. The Way of Adidam is based, from the beginning, on Avatar Adi Da's "Bright" State, Which is Realized progressively (and, ultimately, most perfectly), by means of His Divine Spiritual Descent in the body-mind of His devotee.

18. Avatar Adi Da describes the entire course of practice in the Way of Adidam as falling into four primary phases:

1. listening to Him

2. hearing Him

3. seeing Him

4. the "Perfect Practice" of Identifying with Him

For a description of the unfolding phases of practice of Adidam, see *Adidam: The True World-Religion Given by the Promised God-Man, Adi Da Samraj* and *The Dawn Horse Testament Of The Ruchira Avatar.*

"Listening" is Avatar Adi Da's technical term for the beginning practice of the Way of Adidam. A listening devotee literally "listens" to Avatar Adi Da's Instruction and applies it in his or her life.

The core of the listening process (and of all future practice of the Way of Adidam) is the practice of Ruchira Avatara Bhakti Yoga (or turning the four principal faculties of the body-mind—body, emotion, mind, and breath—to Him)—supported by practice of the "conscious process" and "conductivity" and by the embrace of the functional, practical, relational, and cultural disciplines Given by Him.

It is during the listening phase (once the foundation practice is fully established) that the devotee applies to come on extended formal retreat in Avatar Adi Da's physical Company (or, after His physical Lifetime, in the physical company, and the by-Him-Spiritually-Empowered circumstances, of the Ruchira Sannyasin Order of Adidam Ruchiradam). In the retreat circumstance, when the rightly prepared devotee truly (whole bodily) turns the principal faculties to Him, Avatar Adi Da is spontaneously Moved to Grant His Spiritual Initiation (or Ruchira Shaktipat), such that the devotee can become more and more consistently capable of tangibly receiving His Spiritual Transmission. This is the beginning of the Spiritually Awakened practice of the Way of Adidam—when the devotional relationship to Avatar Adi Da becomes (by His

Divine Spiritual Grace) the devotional-and-Spiritual relationship to Him. The phase of listening to Avatar Adi Da, rightly and effectively engaged, eventually culminates (by His Divine Spiritual Grace) in the true hearing of Him. The devotee has begun to hear Avatar Adi Da when there is most fundamental understanding of the root-act of egoity (or self-contraction), or the unique capability to consistently transcend the self-contraction. The capability of true hearing is not something the ego can "achieve". That capability can only be Granted, by Means of Avatar Adi Da's Divine Spiritual Grace, to His devotee who has effectively completed the (eventually, Spiritually Awakened) process of listening.

When Spiritually Awakened practice of the Way of Adidam is magnified by means of the hearing-capability, the devotee has the necessary preparation to (in due course) engage that Spiritually Awakened practice in the "fully technically responsible" manner. This is another point (in the course of the Way of Adidam) when the devotee engages an extended formal retreat in Avatar Adi Da's physical Company (or, after His physical Lifetime, in the physical company, and the by-Him-Spiritually-Empowered circumstances, of the Ruchira Sannyasin Order of Adidam Ruchiradam). In this case, in Response to the devotee's more mature practice of devotional and Spiritual resort to Him, Avatar Adi Da Gives the Initiatory Spiritual Gift of Upward-turned Spiritual receptivity of Him (as He describes in His "Hridaya Rosary" of "Four Thorns Of Heart-Instruction"). This is Avatar Adi Da's Spiritual Initiation of His devotee into the seeing phase of practice, which Avatar Adi Da describes as the "fully technically responsible" form of Spiritually Awakened resort to Him.

One of the principal signs of the transition from the listening-hearing practice to the both-hearing-and-seeing practice is emotional conversion from the reactive emotions that characterize egoic self-obsession, to the open-hearted, Radiant Happiness that characterizes fully technically responsible Spiritual devotion to Avatar Adi Da. This true and stable emotional conversion coincides with stable Upward-to-Him-turned receptivity of Avatar Adi Da's Spiritual Transmission.

As the process of seeing develops, the body-mind becomes more and more fully Infused by Avatar Adi Da's Spirit-Baptism, purified of any psycho-physical patterning that diminishes that reception. With increasing maturity in the seeing process, Avatar Adi Da's Transmission of the "Bright" is experienced in the unique form that He describes as the "Samadhi of the 'Thumbs'"—and, through this process, the devotee is gracefully grown entirely beyond identification with the body-mind. The seeing process is complete when the devotee receives Avatar Adi Da's Gift of Spiritually Awakening as the Witness-Consciousness (That Stands Prior to body, mind, and world, and even the act of attention itself). This Awakening to the Witness-Consciousness marks readiness for another period of Initiatory retreat in Avatar Adi Da's physical Company (or, after His physical Lifetime, in the physical company, and the by-Him-Spiritually-Empowered circumstances, of the Ruchira Sannyasin Order of Adidam Ruchiradam), in which He Spiritually Initiates the devotee into the "Perfect Practice".

19. The initial phase of the formal full practice of the Way of Adidam, in which one adapts to the primary devotional disciplines of the relationship with Adi Da Samraj, and to all the life-disciplines He has Given.

20. "Sattvic" is the adjectival form of the Sanskrit noun "sattva". In the Hindu tradition, "sattva" is the principle of equilibrium (or harmony), one of the three qualities (or "gunas") of conditionally manifested existence—together with inertia (or "tamas") and activity (or "rajas").

21. To the maximum extent possible, the raw foods selected should be organically grown.

22. Oily fruits, seeds, and nuts may also be eaten in the form of raw (cold pressed) oils—for example, olive oil and coconut oil.

23. The effects cooking has on foods are discussed in such works as:

The Sunfood Diet Success System: 36 Lessons in Health Transformation, by David Wolfe (San Diego, Calif.: Maul Brothers Publishing, 6th ed., 2006).

Eating for Beauty: For Women and Men, by David Wolfe (San Diego, Calif.: Maul Brothers Publishing, 2003).

Conscious Eating, by Gabriel Cousens (Berkeley, Calif.: North Atlantic Books, 2000), pp. 563–64.

Health Secrets from Europe, by Paavo O. Airola (New York: Arco Publishing, 1980), pp. 48–50.

24. *The Eating Gorilla Comes in Peace* (new edition forthcoming from the Dawn Horse Press) is Avatar Adi Da's major "Source-Text" on the practices relating to diet and health in the Way of Adidam. A relatively brief summary of Avatar Adi Da's dietary Instruction is also found in chapter 13 of *The Knee Of Listening.*

25. In His "Source-Text" *The Basket Of Tolerance,* Avatar Adi Da has compiled an extensive list of publications that are useful background study relative to "minimum optimum" diet. The books on this list represent a variety of "points of view" and recommended approaches to diet. The inclusion of a title in this list does not mean that the views presented therein are "endorsed" by Avatar Adi Da Samraj, but (rather) that there is something about the contents of the book that is worth considering. Presented here is a small selection of the principal diet-related books listed by Avatar Adi Da in *The Basket Of Tolerance.*

Toxemia Explained, by J. H. Tilden, MD. Originally published in 1935. Reprinted in various editions.

Fasting for Regeneration: The Short Cut, by Julia Seton. Originally published in 1929. Reprinted in various editions.

Fantastic Voyage: Live Long Enough to Live Forever, by Ray Kurzweil and Terry Grossman, MD. (Emmaus, Penn.: Rodale Books, 2004).

Are You Confused?, by Paavo O. Airola (Pheonix, Ariz.: Health Plus Publishers, 1971).

The Sunfood Diet Success System, by David Wolfe (6th edition).

26. Avatar Adi Da has distinguished three basic psycho-physical types (or strategies), which He has called "vital", "peculiar", and

"solid". The "vital" person is oriented to the physical dimension of existence, the "peculiar" person is oriented to the emotional dimension of existence, and the "solid" person is oriented to the mental dimension of existence. (For Avatar Adi Da's extended Instruction relative to these three psycho-physical types, see *The Dawn Horse Testament Of The Ruchira Avatar*.) While every individual is characteristically dominated by one of these three strategies, the three strategies are not mutually exclusive, and a combination of two or more strategies may need to be taken into account in modifying the diet.

27. Avatar Adi Da describes how one's adaptation to the "minimum optimum" diet must be fully in place to transition beyond the student-beginner stage of the Way of Adidam. However, the "minimum optimum" diet is, by design, always purifying and rejuventating, and, therefore, is constantly and progressively refined as one advances in the Spiritual process altogether.

28. The recipe for the basic "de la Torre" drink is as follows:

Wash but do not peel the following vegetables and cut them into small cubes. Put them into a jar with 6 cups of spring water, if possible, to leach out the water-soluble vitamins and minerals.

> 6 oz. carrots
> 4 oz. beets
> 2 oz. celery
> 2 leaves peppermint

Let the vegetables soak 3–6 hours or overnight in the refrigerator, stirring once or twice. Strain out one cup at a time, as needed, leaving the vegetables in the jar. When there are one or two glasses of liquid left, add one more glass of water to dilute it. You can warm it up on cold days. [From *The Process of Physical Purification by Means of the New and Easy Way to Fast: An Extraordinary, Transcendental Discovery in Body Purification, Showing an Easy and Fast Way to a Higher Degree of Health and Longer Span of Life*, by Teofilo de la Torre (Costa Rica: 1957), pp. 74–78.]

29. The intensive listening-hearing stage of the Way of Adidam begins once a student-beginner has been acknowledged to have reached maturity in the establishment of all the basic life-disciplines of Adidam, and demonstrates the equanimity of concentrated devotional beholding of Adi Da Samraj and sensitivity to His Spiritual Presence. This stage continues until the individual is acknowledged to be "hearing" Avatar Adi Da Samraj (or consistently capable of most fundamental self-understanding).

30. Dairy products, eggs, or flesh foods that are taken upon proper medical advisement should be organic, to the maximum degree possible.

31. Among the life-disciplines Avatar Adi Da gives to His devotees is "cooperative cultural association" with other practitioners of Adidam for the sake of intensified practice and mutual "expectation and inspiration".

32. Examples of such "token and merely symbolic use, as may sometimes be required by custom for respectful and right participation in, necessarily rare, sacred, or entirely ceremonial and non-personal, social occasions" include (perhaps) drinking a small amount of alcohol (or even simply touching one's lips to the liquid) as part of a formal toast at a formal event such as a wedding, smoking a small amount of tobacco at a formal Native American peace pipe ceremony, or drinking a small amount of kava in a formal kava ceremony in the South Pacific.

33. Although fish is the most "sattvic" of flesh foods, care must be taken to avoid fish contaminated with heavy metals and other toxins.

34. If coffee is used as an unavoidable necessity to help alertness, it should be organically grown, to the maximum degree possible.

35. The differences in types of tea are due primarily to differences in the mode of processing the tea leaves after harvesting. In the case of black tea and oolong tea, the processing includes a period of fermentation (or oxidation)—longer in the case of black tea,

shorter in the case of oolong tea. In the case of green tea and white tea, the processing does not include fermentation.

36. Sanskrit word meaning "duty" or "law"—in its fullest sense, refers to living of the Divine Law. A great Spiritual Teaching, including its disciplines and practices can thus be referred to as "Dharma".

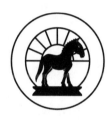

THE DAWN HORSE PRESS

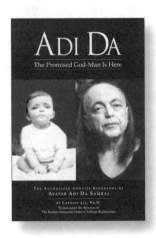

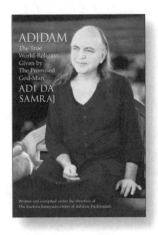

ADI DA
*The Promised God-Man
Is Here*

The biography of Avatar Adi Da
from His Birth to present time.
Includes a wealth of quotations
from His Writings and Talks,
as well as stories told by His
devotees.

358 pp., **$16.95**

ADIDAM
*The True World-Religion
Given by the Promised
God-Man, Adi Da Samraj*

A direct and simple summary of
the fundamental aspects of the
Way of Adidam.

196 pp., **$16.95**

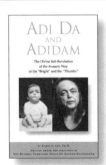

ADI DA AND ADIDAM
*The Divine Self-Revelation
of the Avataric Way of
the "Bright" and the "Thumbs"*

A brief introduction to Avatar Adi Da Samraj
and His Unique Spiritual Revelation of the
Way of Adidam. 64 pp., **$3.95**

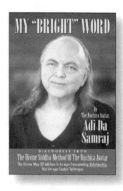

MY "BRIGHT" WORD
by Adi Da Samraj

New Edition of the Classic Spiritual
Discourses originally published as
The Method of the Siddhas

In these Talks from His early Teaching Years,
Avatar Adi Da Gives extraordinary Instruction
on the foundation of True Spiritual life, cover-
ing topics such as the primary mechanism by
which we are preventing the Realization of
Truth, the means to overcome this mechanism, and the true function
of the Spiritual Master in relation to the devotee.

*In modern language, this volume teaches the ancient all-time
trans-egoic truths. It transforms the student by paradox and by
example. Consciousness, understanding, and finally the awakened
Self are the rewards. What more can anyone want?*

—ELMER GREEN, PhD
Director Emeritus, Center for Applied Psychophysiology,
The Menninger Clinic

544 pp., **$24.95**

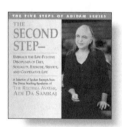

THE FIVE STEPS OF ADIDAM: STEP TWO
Embrace the Life-Positive Disciplines of Diet, Sexuality, Exercise, Service, and Cooperative Life

Excerpts from Talks Given by Avatar Adi Da
that focus on the functional and relational
practices and disciplines that transform every
aspect of daily living into the Yoga of heart-Communion with the
Living Divine Reality. This CD complements the book *Adidam: The
True World-Religion Given by the Promised God-Man, Adi Da Samraj.*

CD, 10 Tracks
Total Running Time: 62 minutes
$16.95

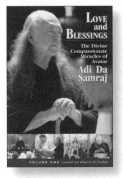

LOVE AND BLESSINGS

The Divine Compassionate Miracles of Avatar Adi Da Samraj

In *Love and Blessings—The Divine Compassionate Miracles of Avatar Adi Da Samraj*, twenty-five of His devotees tell heart-breaking stories of human need and Divine Response. A soldier in Iraq, a woman going blind in Holland, a son with his dying father in Australia, a woman with cancer in America—these and others tell how they asked Adi Da Samraj for His Blessing-Regard and the miraculous process that ensued.

248 pp., **$19.95**

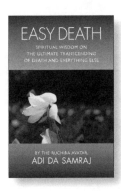

EASY DEATH

Spiritual Wisdom on the Ultimate Transcending of Death and Everything Else
by Adi Da Samraj

This new edition of *Easy Death* is thoroughly revised and updated with:

- New Talks and Essays from Avatar Adi Da on death and ultimate transcendence
- Accounts of profound Events of Yogic Death in Avatar Adi Da's own Life
- Stories of His Blessing in the death transitions of His devotees

. . . an exciting, stimulating, and thought-provoking book that adds immensely to the ever-increasing literature on the phenomena of life and death. But, more important, perhaps, it is a confirmation that a life filled with love instead of fear can lead to ultimately meaningful life and death.

Thank you for this masterpiece.

—ELISABETH KÜBLER-ROSS, MD
author, *On Death and Dying*

544 pp., **$24.95**

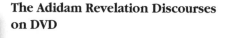

The Adidam Revelation Discourses on DVD

In July of 2004, Adi Da Samraj began a series of Discourses that were broadcast live over the internet to all His devotees around the world. During these remarkable occasions, Adi Da Samraj answered questions from those who were present in the room with Him, but also from devotees in other parts of the world via speakerphone. The "Adidam Revelation Discourse" DVDs offer you the opportunity to see and hear Avatar Adi Da speak in these unique and intimate occasions of Divine Instruction to His devotees. Current available titles include:

TRANSCEND THE SELF-KNOT OF FEAR

Running time: 60 minutes. Includes subtitles in English, Spanish, French, German, Dutch, and Polish.

THE DIVINE IS NOT THE CAUSE

Running time: 72 minutes. Includes subtitles in English, Spanish, French, German, Dutch, Finnish, Polish, Czech, Chinese, Japanese, and Hebrew.

CRACKING THE CODE OF EXPERIENCE

Running time: 86 minutes. Includes subtitles in English, Spanish, German, Dutch, Polish, Czech, Chinese, Japanese, and Hebrew.

DVD, **$26.95** each.

To find out about and order other "Source-Texts", books, tapes, CDs, DVDs, and videos by and about Avatar Adi Da, contact your local Adidam regional center, or contact the Dawn Horse Press at:

1-877-770-0772 (from within North America)
1-707-928-6653 (from outside North America)
Or order online from: **www.dawnhorsepress.com**

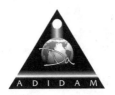

We invite you to find out more about Avatar Adi Da Samraj and the Way of Adidam

■ Find out about our courses, seminars, events, and retreats by calling the regional center nearest you.

AMERICAS
12040 N. Seigler Rd.
Middletown, CA
95461 USA
1-707-928-4936

THE UNITED KINGDOM
uk@adidam.org
0845-330-1008

EUROPE-AFRICA
Annendaalderweg 10
6105 AT Maria Hoop
The Netherlands
31 (0)20 468 1442

PACIFIC-ASIA
12 Seibel Road
Henderson
Auckland 1008
New Zealand
64-9-838-9114

AUSTRALIA
P.O. Box 244
Kew 3101
Victoria
**1800 ADIDAM
(1800-234-326)**

INDIA
Shree Love-Ananda Marg
Rampath, Shyam Nagar Extn.
Jaipur–302 019, India
91 (141) 2293080

E-MAIL: **correspondence@adidam.org**

■ Order books, tapes, CDs, DVDs, and videos by and about Avatar Adi Da Samraj.

1-877-770-0772 (from within North America)
1-707-928-6653 (from outside North America)
order online: **www.dawnhorsepress.com**

■ Visit us online:

www.adidam.org

Explore the online community of Adidam and discover more about Avatar Adi Da and the Way of Adidam.